"*Deep Medicine* offers a free-spirited approach to exploring your innate health-building potential."

—Mehmet Oz, MD, heart surgeon and coauthor of
YOU: The Owner's Manual

"When it comes to our health, our choices are often our destiny. In *Deep Medicine,* Dr. Stewart supports our choices with the skill of a surgeon and the wisdom of a healer."

—Rachel Naomi Remen, MD, professor and author of
Kitchen Table Wisdom

"Dr. Stewart is a pioneer in holistic and mind-body medicine and was one of the first clinicians in America to build a firm bridge between holistic and conventional medicine."

—Larry Dossey, MD, author of *Healing Words* and
The Power of Premonitions

"Dr. Stewart has pioneered a new and effective approach to body/mind/ spirit healing."

—Justine and Michael Toms, cofounders of New Dimensions
World Broadcasting Network and coauthors of *True Work*

"In a most magical way, Dr. Stewart shares what he has learned about life and living well. Readers will be engaged and discover that their personal wellness is connected with everyone and everything."

—Bob Duggan, MA, M.Ac., president of The Tai Sophia
Institute in Laurel, MD

deep
medicine

harnessing the source of your healing power

William B. Stewart, MD

Noetic Books, Institute of Noetic Sciences
New Harbinger Publications, Inc.

Publisher's Note

Distributed in Canada by Raincoast Books

A copublication of New Harbinger Publications and Noetics Books.

Copyright © 2009 by William B. Stewart
New Harbinger Publications, Inc.
5674 Shattuck Avenue
Oakland, CA 94609
www.newharbinger.com

Acquired by Jess O'Brien; Cover design by Amy Shoup; Cover photograph: Datura H, © Doris Mitsch; Edited by Jasmine Star; Text design by Tracy Marie Carlson

Library of Congress Cataloging-in-Publication Data

Stewart, William B. (William Bennett), 1943-
 Deep medicine : harnessing the source of your healing power / William B. Stewart ; foreword by Angeles Arrien.
     p. cm.
 Includes bibliographical references.
 ISBN-13: 978-1-57224-644-7 (pbk. : alk. paper)
 ISBN-10: 1-57224-644-8 (pbk. : alk. paper)
 1.   Health--Philosophy. 2.   Self-care, Health.
3. Mind and body. 4.
Healing. 5. Spirituality. I. Title.
RA776.5.S8146 2009
613--dc22
                                    2009014651

FSC
Mixed Sources
Product group from well-managed
forests and other controlled sources

Cert no. SW-COC-002283
www.fsc.org
© 1996 Forest Stewardship Council

11 10 09
10 9 8 7 6 5 4 3 2 1   First printing

With deep respect and gratitude, this book is dedicated to Dr. Govindappa Venkataswamy (Dr. V), who, through his and his family's vision and mission at the Aravind Eye Hospitals in India, showed me the possibilities of braiding science, service, and spirit in the practice of medicine; to Angeles Arrien, Ph.D., whose cross-cultural synthesis of principles and practices for health and healing provides access to the language and tools to manifest deep medicine; and to my life partner, Susy Stewart, whose gifts, talents, and love are daily blessings.

Contents

Foreword

Cross-culturally, the power of choice for human beings has three functions: First, through choice we can create a new experience or reality for ourselves that inspires us. Second, through choice we can end an experience or reality for ourselves that is no longer tolerable. And third, through choice we can maintain and sustain our current experience or reality as it is.

Often these choices present themselves during times of change and transition. Most people tend to support the third function: what is knowable, comfortable, and controllable. However, when we are healthy and happy, we're motivated and tend to gravitate to the first function: making choices that support what has heart and meaning. And if we can no longer tolerate the experience or reality we've created, we will choose the second option: to galvanize our actions to create change. What choices are we making that are currently health creating? What choices are we making that are health negating?

In a time when obesity, heart disease, cancer, and diabetes are at their highest rates, *Deep Medicine* provides a necessary and very palatable antidote for reducing illness and disease and enhancing well-being in our lives. How we engage in the four pillars of self-care offered in this book—nutrition, physical activity and relaxation, relationship and community, and contemplation and solitude—on a daily basis determines the sustainability of our health and healing. By engaging in our own self-care, we can truly become primary care physicians for ourselves.

As the medical director of the Institute for Health and Healing at California Pacific Medical Center in San Francisco, Dr. William Stewart successfully practices and advocates a holistic approach to health and healing that combines contemporary medicine with a worldview that acknowledges the complexity of the ingredients contributing to our well-being, or our lack of it. Dr. Stewart's most compelling message is "Everything is either health creating or health negating. Everything!" According to Dr. Stewart, everything we think, feel, say, and do contributes to our health. Seeing health from this truly holistic perspective motivates us to make choices that serve personal wellness and then go further, to contribute to enduring public health and aid planetary healing.

Every day provides a new canvas on which to create health. *Deep Medicine* offers complete and thorough guidance on both practical and universal ways in which we can change our health and well-being internally and externally, mentally and emotionally, and physically and spiritually. The human spirit is always reaching for the reclamation of its own well-being. *Deep Medicine* offers a compelling invitation into a process and a way of thinking by which we can choose to make that our experience and our reality.

Dr. Stewart remains the foremost advocate and guide on this transformative, evolutionary healing path that empowers responsible health care and health-creating choices. *Deep Medicine* reminds us that eradicating disease, creating health, and preventing future illness are personal and collective sacred tasks. If we accept the premise that we have a responsibility for our own health and well-being, then it follows that we are all healers.

Deep Medicine is an outstanding contribution to the fields of integrative medicine and preventive medicine—and medicine in general. Dr. Stewart's call to each of us as a doctor and a healer is to actively engage our health and well-being using the concepts, tools, and practices in this book. Will we be conscious of the choices we are making and committed to the changes we desire? Let us begin our holy healing work and choose health for ourselves, others, and the world.

—Angeles Arrien, cultural anthropologist

Acknowledgments

The manifestation of this version of *Deep Medicine: Harnessing the Source of Your Healing Power* rests on the shoulders of those who contributed to planting the seeds and nurturing the sprout of the first incarnation, and some important others who saw a potential for enhancing the original and making *Deep Medicine* available to a new and larger audience.

My thanks to Matthew Gilbert, director of communications at the Institute of Noetic Sciences, and to editor Jess O'Brien at New Harbinger Publications, who opened the conversation and trusted in the worth of this project.

I am indebted to Beth Witrogen, who brought her considerable editing skills and creative expression to subtracting what needed to be eliminated and adding to what needed more substance. Doug Winger helped simplify, clarify, and interpret the promise of *Deep Medicine*. Copy editor Jasmine Star brought her gentle touch to aligning and refining the final product. Milena Fiore, fine nurse and caregiver that she is, helped maintain the balance between my "day job" and the revision and renewal of *Deep Medicine*. Their caring interventions were well tolerated by the "patient," who became stronger in the process. Thanks are also due to Doris Mitsch for the cover art, and for her many gifts and talents.

I am grateful to my colleagues, the staff, and our patients and supporters at the Institute for Health and Healing (IHH), and to Drs. Bruce Spivey and Martin Brotman, CEOs at the California Pacific Medical Center, San Francisco, for their support during the genesis and evolution of IHH. Judith Tolson has been a gifted leader at the IHH since its inception. Without her capacity to manifest a transformative vision of healing and her enduring encouragement, both IHH and *Deep Medicine* might still be on a to-do list waiting to happen.

The patience, understanding, and support of my family during the many hours I spent writing this book provided the needed sustenance for the journey and many lasting lessons in my personal practice of deep medicine.

INTRODUCTION

Bridging Science and Spirit

If you are looking for the greatest treasure, don't look outside. Look within. Seek that.

—Rumi

There is no happiness that is not somehow rooted in the task of systematic self-examination.

—Plato

Everything you think, feel, say, and do is either health creating or health negating. Everything.

Whether you're talking about the symptoms of a heart attack or stroke, or findings related to diabetes or a diagnosis of cancer; whether you're talking about environmental degradation, social injustice, economic disparity, poverty, violence, or spiritual crisis—you're talking about health issues in some way. There is nothing that isn't related to the state of our personal and collective well-being. Therefore, every issue is a health issue.

Your personal health depends on what you think, how you feel, and how you act. It also depends on your habits, your values, your choices, your character, your sense of purpose, and the meaning you bring to your life. Health necessitates proper nutrition, appropriate physical activity and rest, contemplation and solitude, and the support of relationships and community. You are healthy when you are in a state of balance and equilibrium regarding your bodily processes and in relationship to your surroundings. When you lose this balance, you become ill and healing is needed.

Deep Medicine is a book about bringing your external and internal resources together for health-creating change and to foster well-being and healing. It is about awakening your inner healer and harnessing your own healing power.

SEEDS OF SERVICE

In 1983, I visited India for the first time. There I had the privilege of working at the Aravind Eye Hospital in Madurai, an institution that is the result of the pioneering work of Dr. Govindappa Venkataswamy. From that time forward, my life as both a surgeon and a human being was permanently transformed.

After his retirement in 1976 as the chair of the Department of Ophthalmology at the nearby medical school, Dr. V, as he was lovingly called, was moved by a desire to serve his community with a higher standard of ophthalmic care, regardless of caste or capacity to pay. He opened a small eye hospital in a converted house with two operating rooms and twelve beds.

From this humble beginning, and with the help of Dr. V's dedicated family, the organization has become the world's largest eye care system. Presently more than 1.5 million patients are cared for and more than 250,000 surgeries are performed annually at five hospitals. What makes this even more remarkable is that approximately two-thirds of the treatments are done on a "free hospital" basis. That is, each patient who is able to pay supports two who cannot. The work is of the highest quality, performed to international standards and accomplished within a balanced budget.

Dr. V, a physically slight man with fingers gnarled from severe inflammatory arthritis that afflicted him from a young age, lived authentically and with a burning passion to fight needless blindness, along with a vision of how to do it. He was a healer of giant proportion, a surgeon who lived fully in the worlds of both science and spirit and a mentor and role model to many. The purpose of his life and the meaning of his existence remain clearly evident in his healing legacy. His life and his work seamlessly integrated deep spiritual practice with compassionate service in the secular world. In the presence of his own illness, he lived a life of health and healing.

At the Aravind Eye Hospital, I discovered a place where science and spirit are yoked in a model that embodies a collaborative healing relationship between scientific expertise and spiritual richness— between medicine and meaning. It is a bridge where the truths of science meet the truths of the sacred, and where the practical, purposeful, and paradoxical come together. Underlying the bustle of busy operating rooms (often with two or three surgeries occurring simultaneously) and the chaos of crowded corridors is a reverence for every being. There the staff exhibits a deep, powerful connection to an unseen inner energy reservoir—a spirit of service and purpose that moves many of them to begin each day in the hospital's meditation room.

It was on that first trip to India that the seeds of deep medicine were planted. It was there that I saw in practice that health and healing are not just scientific but also spiritual pursuits, where both visible (external) and invisible (inner) worlds play an active, collaborative role.

TAKING MEDICINE TO HEART

I went to India as a young, well-trained surgeon full of the desire to help those needing and doing ophthalmic surgery in the developing world. I returned humbled by the volume and quality of the work being done, deeply moved by the compassion demonstrated, inspired by the generosity of spirit I saw, and changed by the joy that emanated from the deeply committed people I met. The dedication, compassion, and skillful medical care that I witnessed there changed my perspective on the practice of medicine, as well as my understanding of health and healing.

Early in my career, I believed that living a healthy life was the responsibility of the individual, but that healing disease was the responsibility of a doctor. Over the past forty years, these views have shifted. As I have grown as a surgeon and a person, I have come to realize that the state of one's health impacts every aspect of his or her life, from work to worries and from behaviors to beliefs. I have seen patients expected to die make miraculous recoveries while others succumb for no discernible reason.

By definition, "medicine" means the art and science of healing; a remedy, potion, or drug; possessing or controlling power; and a deserved punishment. Its formal practice ranges from environmental medicine to forensic medicine to geriatric care; from socialized to tropical to veterinary; and from traditional to alternative, indigenous, unorthodox, complementary, mind-body, multidimensional, preventive, integrative, and simply "good" medicine. The profession has many nuances, nooks, and crannies as it seeks to reduce and relieve pain and suffering, to cure disease, and to heal illness.

Oftentimes medical issues are so objectified that they aren't seen in a holistic way. For example, if you're afflicted with pain, you may have arthritis in a joint, an ulcer in your stomach, or an infection in your bladder. However, there are also aspects of illness that may live deeper within; these might be called the substance beneath the symptoms. Consider this inner landscape as the region of your thoughts, your emotions, your reactions, your dreams, your desires, your fears, and the mythological or spiritual realm within—your very being. These aspects of health and disease are often neither recognized nor attended to with the same rigor as the outer landscape. Yet they can be responsible for sickness, too.

A HOLISTIC HEALING PROCESS

I see healing as a deep and mysterious process. A process much more complex than can be explained by anatomy, physiology, and pathology alone. An intricate interplay of genetics, environment, fate, destiny, thoughts, emotions, story, conditioning, and luck that often defies clear alignment between cause and effect.

In the early 1990s, as part of my quest to more fully understand health and healing, and to attempt to bring aspects of the holistic approach I saw in India into established medical practice in the United States, I cofounded the Institute for Health and Healing (IHH) at California Pacific Medical Center in San Francisco. Today it is recognized as a national leader in evidence-based integrative medicine, combining knowledge bases, skill sets, and practices from other cultures and other times with contemporary medicine. Staffed with board-certified physicians and licensed practitioners, IHH bridges science and the sacred, with an emphasis on relationship-centered care. At the institute, self-care and expert care are combined in an ongoing collaboration in classes, support groups, retreats, workshops, in-hospital and outpatient care, and basic and clinical research. The program includes traditional Chinese medicine, ayurvedic practices from India, nutritional consultation and counseling, art therapy, guided imagery, massage therapy, yoga, meditation, tai chi and qigong, Pilates, and Feldenkrais. Most significantly perhaps, the hospital chaplaincy is also a part of IHH. This allows the institute to actually manifest the often-described holistic health triad of caring for body, mind, and spirit. The institute's success in serving more than fifty thousand people each year is the reason California Pacific Medical Center was named America's Healthiest Hospital by *Natural Health* magazine in 2001 (Gallia 2001).

My years as a surgeon have taught me that we cannot deal with illness without dealing with the spiritual aspects of illness any more than we can deal with illness without dealing with its genetic implications. Although our genes aren't necessarily seen and we don't feel them, they underlie much of our health status. The work of deep medicine seeks to go beyond medicine to combine health care practices from the best of contemporary, biotechnical medicine with more spiritual and inner aspects of healing—aspects like caring, compassion, and purpose, as well as the management of contributors to disease, such as stress, emotions, and resistance to change.

Balancing these many aspects of life leads to health. Your work toward health and healing is not only physical work toward living better, but also soul work toward self-realization: being in the present, accepting paradox, and choosing wisely. These are the tools you will explore in *Deep Medicine*.

WHY DEEP MEDICINE?

Deep medicine connects your personal health with everything that surrounds you. It integrates simple techniques with recognition of the need for lifelong learning and practice so th at you can create your own optimal path to health. It is this integration that provides the greatest potential for meaningful, lasting, and truly transformative living.

All issues are health issues, and in order to engage your health issues, it's necessary to go inward. The term "deep" in the book's title means below the surface, not superficial; learned, wise, and within. In the context of this book, it also means profound, heartfelt, sincere, intense, great in measure, and mysterious. The term "medicine" implies the power of healing; when applied specifically, it can become your own system for creating better personal health.

Deep medicine isn't a surface paint job; it's a new foundation. It isn't a perfumed cover-up; it's a deep cleansing. The work of creating health and healing is a personal, lifelong, and conscious process that must examine the inner depths as well as refine surface contours. Just like the sign frequently seen in office windows instructs—"Help Wanted, Inquire Within"—in order to practice deep medicine you must inquire within and then act on what you learn.

It is this inner quest for your personal truth that awakens the healer within, harnesses your personal sources of healing power, and supports health and healing in the fullest way. Learning to slow down and become present and quiet starts this work. Focusing your attention and intention and going inward moves it forward. This can be begun by simply treating yourself to a moment of quiet contemplation, reflection, and grounding through use of the "deep minute" (see chapter 4).

Deep Medicine: Harnessing the Source of Your Healing Power looks beneath the superficiality of symptoms to the underlying issues of health. It explores the complex, interwoven nature of health as part of the immense mystery of life rather than reducing it to an easily explainable puzzle to be hastily solved. Our bodies should not be treated like machines that can be fixed by merely changing a part or using a standard healing process. Without deeper inquiry and self-discovery, approaches to well-being will likely fall short of promised results and will also be unsustainable. This book's perspectives and practices will continue to foster self-discovery, self-efficacy, and self-directed healing long after many of the popular health trends of today have faded from memory.

Deep Medicine is steeped in principles of integrative medicine, an approach that is both multidisciplinary and relationship centered. That is, it educates and empowers individuals to be active participants in their own care while drawing on expert care for the broadest understanding of the nature of health, illness, and healing. It is based on a holistic approach to the health and healing of mind, body, and spirit in the context of the collective and the community—and the planet.

Deep medicine has a strong link to ancient and timeless medical knowledge and practices. Keeping this healing heritage alive and honoring past contributions from many sources has the potential to strengthen contemporary medicine as new knowledge and practices are discovered (and rediscovered) over coming decades.

Deep medicine honors each person's individual story and understands that emotion can override reason. Deep medicine recognizes that the pace of contemporary life makes it difficult to find time to reflect, contemplate, and integrate. It makes use of a broad spectrum of evidence-based therapies from multiple cultures to support the creation of personal well-being, public health, and global healing across the life span and across cultures.

What you really need to know about creating health is not only how to start the specific tasks of a valuable wellness or healing program, but especially how to sustain the demanding work. Even when you're under the care of an expert, your lifestyle choices continue to have a tremendous impact on your state of well-being and your healing progress. You and your doctor cannot merely prescribe, order, or wish health or healing any more than you can mandate happiness or demand creativity. What you *can* do is establish the cornerstones, plot the course, and gather the tools for healthy living. Ultimately, you need to build and to trust your own experience. You need to do your own insightful thinking, planning, and prioritizing, and then commit to action.

But you don't have to do it alone.

For me, the seeds of deep medicine were planted in India, and they germinated at the Institute for Health and Healing, with its superb staff and the many people who have used the extensive intake questionnaire to assess their symptoms, attitudes, motivation, and progress toward goals. (This assessment is condensed in the exercises at the end of chapter 1.) Our practitioners' experience led the institute to develop a basic yet sustainable integrative approach. At the heart of this approach is the realization that a self-defined personal program is the one most likely to be adhered to and thus lead to sustainable results.

The program you create for yourself is the one most likely to succeed for you. This book will guide you along the path of creating such a program. It only takes a minute to begin to realize and harness your healing power, and with time, you can expand your skills into a rich lifestyle of wellness practices and better health. Through the practice of deep medicine, you will learn how to do all of the following, and more:

ꕥ Value and enhance your inner wisdom and resources as actively as your outer resources in the pursuit of health and healing.

ꕥ Align your deepest knowing with your everyday actions.

- Be fully present to yourself and others.

- Develop your character.

- Use the deep minute as part of your self-care.

- Balance service to others with service to yourself.

- Consider the greater good and the long view in all of your thoughts, decisions, and actions.

FOUR CORNERSTONES

Deep Medicine is based on four foundational cornerstones:

1. **Four questions of self-assessment** that provide a way to take your "vital signs" without a blood-pressure cuff or a scale—or six months alone on a desert island (chapter 1)

2. **Four core competencies** that support the process of change and help build character and sustainable habits (chapters 2 and 3)

3. **Four pillars of self-care**, common practices of health and healing that contribute to well-being (covered in chapter 4)

4. **Four practices** that facilitate contact with and development of the healer within (also covered in chapter 4)

Chapters 5 through 7 give guidance for deepening the inner work of health creation, and then expand the meaning of health beyond the personal to the planetary while helping you define your unique healing story. Your dynamic story will serve to sustain a lifetime of wellness practices and help you come to terms with the many paradoxical pairs that populate the world of health and healing, such as body and spirit, science and soul, emotion and reason, need and want, pain and pleasure, and sadness and joy.

Initiating and sustaining health-creating change is not a sprint; it's a marathon. Whether you are facing an acute health crisis, coping with a life-threatening illness or chronic condition, or seeking general well-being, peak performance, or optimal aging, you can use *Deep Medicine* as a handbook for creating a healthier life. Although there is no fixed, one-size-fits-all formula for healing or for creating health, progress does tend to occur in sequence, with each advance building on the previous one and setting the stage for the next. This book offers practical exercises for outer lifestyle changes, and also helps you learn how to engage your inner resources so you can successfully negotiate the many choices and decisions necessary for vital health. These negotiations must lead to conclusions that are aligned with the meaning and purpose of your life, or they will evaporate. Since all issues are health issues, *Deep Medicine* also offers a mix of philosophy and practical skills applicable in some way to almost every key issue you will confront in life.

The exercises that conclude chapters 1 through 6 are meant to encourage progress on your path of self-inquiry and discovery. There are no right or wrong answers. Asking and holding thought-provoking questions is more important. This methodology is both challenging— to honestly examine your behaviors and beliefs—and empowering, since you gain insights into how to choose for health. You don't need to answer all of the questions at once. Take small steps. Address a specific area of interest. Look for one or two approaches that speak to you about lending balance to your life and try them. Build patiently from there.

You might consider using a notebook or journal to complete the exercises and record your answers, raise your own questions, and track your course. In this way, you will write your own book of health.

YOU ARE IN THE DRIVER'S SEAT

My car is parked in the parking lot. There is only one key, and I've got it. As you look at your health, grateful that the body you are blessed to be in is your vehicle, you'll appreciate that *you* have the key to it—and that you need to accept the responsibility of being in the driver's seat. If in the course of driving you hear a strange noise, experience erratic steering, cannot slow your speed or control your direction, are still in darkness when you turn on the lights, or see a warning light on the dashboard go on, don't turn up the radio and ignore the signs of trouble or take the car to a car wash. As my colleague Dr. Michael Cantwell of the Institute for Health and Healing is fond of saying, you have to look under the hood. Once you do, be prepared to make the needed repair or, if it is beyond your capacity to do so, seek expert help. You have to go inward to look deeper. To do so, you have to be prepared and willing to fully assess the situation by slowing down, being quiet, coming present, and opening to your inner wisdom with focused attention and intention.

When you can do that, you are practicing deep medicine.

From our external physical boundaries to the limitless expanse of our inner landscape, understanding health requires keeping some basic concepts in mind:

- ❧ The essence of personal health is holistic. Even as we acknowledge the external and physical aspects of health and disease, we must also recognize the nonmaterial and inner aspects of creating health.

- ❧ Everything you think, feel, say, and do is either health creating or health negating. Every issue is a health issue.

- ❧ The basic building block of health and healing is relationship: to self, to intimate others, to community, to the planet, and to the sacred and spiritual aspects of life.

- ❧ Personal transformation—a deep philosophic shift—is often necessary if health-creating life choices are to be lasting and sustainable.

- ❧ The core challenge is how to go about changing. Leaving your comfort zone is necessary in this endeavor.

- ❧ Learning to be in the present moment is important, since it's the only place where you can really make choices.

- ❧ Because creating health demands authenticity, commitment, discipline, honesty, integrity, and trust, among other essential traits, it requires the development of character.

- ❧ The driving forces in our collective approach to health care today are primarily economic, political, and scientific.

MOVING FORWARD

Deep Medicine will help you move toward health and healing in a deliberate way. You will forge a dynamic path that develops through successes, learning, and course corrections. After reading *Deep Medicine*, you will have an evolving, transformative, and personal approach to health that will last a lifetime. It is my hope that in creating wellness and balance, you will also discover, or commit more vitally to, the meaning, purpose, and joy in your life—and to the unique gifts you are here to express and to share.

Every day, we are all inundated by images of popular ideas of health and beauty. Quick-fix workout programs, silver bullet pills, and expensive retreats claim to help impatient consumers lose weight and live a healthier life. But many of these remedies are superficial and inadequate. Health is not about how beautiful you look, how old you are, or how big your muscles are. Health is about balance, healing is about change, and both require us to practice deep medicine.

In the words of Dr. Govindappa Venkataswamy, "When we grow in spiritual consciousness, we identify ourselves with all that is in the world. So there is no exploitation. It is ourselves we are helping. It is ourselves we are healing" (2004).

CHAPTER 1

What Is Deep Medicine?

Healing has always been the common meeting ground between the physical and the spiritual. When we experience illness, even something as minor as a cold or the flu, we are brought face to face with our vulnerability, and if we look ahead, which we are prone to do at such moments, we can see death. As a result, illness has always been a breeding ground for spiritual concerns.

—Larry Dossey, MD

The body is your temple. Keep it pure and clean for the soul to reside in.

—B. K. S. Iyengar

One of my earliest childhood memories is pretending to be a doctor as a preschooler, with a toy stethoscope and a clinic of ailing stuffed animals. Not too many years later, this game became reality as I began my medical training.

In the 1960s, while I was in college and medical school, dramatic change was in the air in the world of medicine. Heart surgeons were performing magic at the body's core. Organ transplantation was the new focus for pioneers and visionaries. Imaging equipment that would revolutionize diagnostic capabilities was on the drawing board. New drugs, based on rapidly expanding research efforts, were flooding the marketplace, and government-sponsored health insurance for the elderly—Medicare—was initiated, sparking the fear of socialized medicine in the hearts of established practitioners.

My medical practice began in general surgery training and evolved into highly specialized ophthalmic plastic and reconstructive surgery. I have since become medical director of an institute integrating holistic and conventional practices, with an increasing emphasis on education, leadership, and service. I have operated barefoot in India with handheld flashlights. I've encountered acupuncturists in pain clinics, massage therapists in intensive care units, and chaplains on hospital rounds. I have seen unexplained recoveries from terminal illness, and I've seen people die for no apparent reason. I have come to appreciate how tortuous the path and how complex the contributing factors are to each person's illness and well-being.

I have learned that there is no single, simple path to health. Everything we think, feel, do, and say either creates health or negates it. Furthermore, I have come to believe that every issue is a health issue.

The boundaries of medical practice continue to evolve. We are mapping the human genome and elucidating complex cellular and subcellular physiologic processes, even as practices such as traditional Chinese medicine, ayurveda (the indigenous medicine of India), homeopathy, naturopathy, yoga, and meditation are becoming more widely understood and applied. There are both individual and collective movements toward relationship, collaboration, integration, wholeness, and prevention in today's practice of medicine. This is occurring even as biotechnical, pharmacologic, and genetic breakthroughs are reported almost daily.

Yet estimates of the number of people whose symptoms represent "psychosomatic," "functional," or "stress-mediated" illness continue to be significant. With chronic illness in all age groups on the increase and the population aging, challenges to health care providers are clear and growing. It is understandable that people are seeking integrative or alternative solutions outside mainstream Western medicine and are turning to their own self-care, and it is likely that this will continue to occur in the future.

What can we learn from this paradox of suffering from more disease and illness even while enjoying more scientific and medical advances? One lesson we can learn is that we don't pay enough attention to the meaning and sources of true health. Perhaps we don't appreciate our health until it is compromised or we have lost it. Perhaps we don't appreciate all of the things that influence, both negatively and positively, our health and well-being. What we need to understand about health is its holistic nature, its dependence on aspects of character (for instance honesty, discipline, or patience), and the relationship of the healing journey to the choices we make and the way we live. John Astin, Ph.D., of the California Pacific Medical Center in San Francisco, evaluated why patients use alternative medicine. He pointed out that in alternative therapies patients find "an acknowledgment of the importance of treating illness within a larger context of spirituality and life meaning… The use of alternative care is part of a broader value orientation and set of cultural beliefs, one that embraces a holistic, spiritual orientation to life" (1998, p. 1552).

THE WINDS OF CHANGE

In recent years, a visible change in thinking about health and disease has been occurring. Arenas as seemingly diverse as genetics, nutrition, and self-realization have found themselves fully in the public eye and medical consciousness as they come together in creative ways for medical treatments and new lifestyle approaches. As the public eats broccoli, savors the healthy fats in salmon, and attends stress management classes, new data are appearing in the medical literature supporting the power of lifestyle choices. Recommendations from mainstream institutions such as the American Heart Association, the

American Diabetes Association, the American Cancer Society, and even the National Institutes of Health have accepted therapeutic lifestyle change as a first line of therapy and a standard of care in the management of many conditions (Eyre et al. 2004).

Recently, light has been shed on a constellation of health risk factors known collectively as metabolic syndrome, which is characterized by abdominal obesity and elevated blood pressure, blood lipids, and blood sugar. While it afflicts an estimated 50 million adults, metabolic syndrome is often without symptoms. Metabolic syndrome is important because this combination of risk factors is related to the incidence of cardiovascular disease, stroke, diabetes, and cancer—the most common causes of annual mortality in the United States (Malik et al. 2004). The diseases associated with metabolic syndrome lead to a large percentage of U.S. health care costs. Increasingly, health care plans and employers are looking for ways to reduce the health care cost burden. Because addressing health risk factors can play an important role in reducing these costs, lifestyle change programs are beginning to find a place in mainstream health care practice. Of course, they also bring the more immediate and human benefit of greater health and well-being.

Improving our health depends not just on greater availability of general information about health and healthful lifestyle choices, but also on how people apply this information within the complexity of their own lives and in association with their own genetic individuality and personal preferences. One exciting recent development in this regard is the possibility of optimizing our individual genetic potential. It is also the thrust of a new scientific discipline called nutrigenomics, which inquires into how gene expression is influenced by diet and nutrition (Bland and Benum 1999; Browner et al. 2004). This line of study will likely have strong influence over what and how we eat and how we use supplements in the foreseeable future. Similar lines of inquiry may relate our genetic expression to exercise, attitude and mood, contemplative practice, stress management, and social and relational networks (Ornish et al. 2008).

The medical culture is moving more toward prevention and early detection of disease, and into the realm of actually creating health, rather than focusing on treating symptoms and diseases later in their course (Chopra et al. 2009). As medical practice and the science underlying it continue to develop, new information and recommendations will be forthcoming. Be open to new knowledge and wisdom about how to create your own personal health and well-being. That said, the recommendations and practices in *Deep Medicine* will stand you in good stead. Many of them have already passed the test of time, and many of them have been used by many cultures to create and enhance health.

WHY CHANGE?

The challenges to our health are internal and external, individual and collective. They are genetic, environmental, communal, cultural, physical, infectious, degenerative, inflammatory, mental, and spiritual. These factors are so varied and interwoven that discerning cause and effect can be difficult. Yet attempting to be holistic does not eliminate the need to look at each part—body, mind, and spirit—separately.

As you look at your state of health and well-being, it isn't necessary to find fault or place blame. It is only necessary to honestly be present with what is. To create a healthier future, you must be accountable to yourself and committed to making the most of what you have. Whereas there are things you *can* do about your health, there is much you have no control over. You must move forward from the present time and your current circumstances. No matter what your current health condition is, greater well-being and healing are always possible.

We often know what to do about our health challenges. We are instructed and educated by multiple sources every day. We may even know how to do it. Myriad plans, programs, books, CDs, lectures, workshops, and retreats are available to us.

But do we do what's needed to safeguard and enhance our health? Not usually. It is often more compelling to remember our failures or to worry about what might happen than to act here and now. It is much easier to shop for walking shoes than to use them; to join a yoga class than to attend it regularly; or to buy a book than to read it (and easier to read it than follow its advice). It is noteworthy how many people will use an expensive pharmaceutical or undergo an invasive surgical procedure rather than give up a sedentary lifestyle, change unhealthful eating habits, or forgo addictive behaviors.

Somehow, a wide gap exists between our knowledge about what to do to be healthy and actually acting on that knowledge. Too often it takes a crisis to move us do something about our health: a frightening diagnosis or symptoms we can't ignore. Then, when we realize our problems have become serious, we turn to experts for guidance and care. At that point, it may be too late for preventive measures to affect the state of our health, so only more invasive and "heroic" measures have the potential to change the course of an established disease.

What propels a person to change and what prevents a person from making desired changes? As will be discussed in chapter 2, changing is the true challenge on the path to health and healing. What is really most important regarding your health is not the particular diet plan or exercise program you decide to pursue, but actually doing it! The doing requires a deep, personal evocation of motivation, will, and action and is much more difficult than simply *deciding* what to do. Dedication, discipline, and commitment are among the requirements, as are honesty, flexibility, accountability, responsibility, and patience. These are all character traits. This is where deep medicine comes in, as inspiration and as a guide to the health-creating practices you will learn about in this book—all of which will support lasting change for greater well-being.

WHAT IS HEALTH?
WHAT IS HEALING?

Once, during an invigorating discussion with a group of bright young students, I was asked to define health in one word. After a brief, thoughtful silence, I said, "Balance." A follow-up question quickly surfaced: "If health is balance, then what is healing?" My response was instantaneous: "Change!"

Both definitions form the basis of deep medicine. The word "health" comes from the Indo-European word *kailo*. This root word is the origin of the English words "whole" and "holy," as well as "health." Whereas today our concept of health is typically limited to our physical and mental status, the legacy of the word itself implies something broader—and well it should.

Today's dominant medical model defines diseases and illnesses primarily in physical and epidemiologic terms: bacterial meningitis (infection of brain linings), gastric ulcer (erosion of stomach lining), osteoporosis (loss of density of bone), myocardial infarction (death of the heart muscle). However, to understand the true nature of health, we need to look broadly and deeply at some complex aspects. Even the World Health Organization has defined health not simply as the absence of disease, but as a positive state of physical, mental, and social well-being. In 1984, the World Health Assembly added spiritual health to its definition. More recently, a wealth of solid scientific evidence has come forth supporting the effects on one's state of well-being of such influences as prayer, intention, attitude, beliefs, and social support.

If your understanding of health is limited, you risk being blind to its spiritual, social, and mythological influences. No illness has a single, specific physical cause. Being healthy means more than attaining an ideal weight, having "normal" lab test results, or conforming to the legal definition of sanity. Even when you catch a cold after an airplane trip or during finals week, your illness is more than simply the result of a viral or bacterial source. Stress, fatigue, and dehydration all play a role in your susceptibility. To ignore some of the less obvious factors contributing to your state of health is to have an incomplete picture of the situation—as well as a diminished chance for true healing and well-being.

Your health cannot be easily separated from other major domains of your life: your work and creative purpose; your relationships (to self, intimate others, groups, collectives, nature, and the divine, mystery, or spirit); and your sense of prosperity, resources, abundance, and blessing. Your very existence is often characterized mainly in material terms. You are labeled teacher, parent, student, employee, or friend, names that fail to capture the full grandeur of the human condition, such as your roots, your potential, and the vast interconnectedness in which you exist. You are more than your roles, accomplishments, diagnoses, associations, fears, or mistakes. When you are able to recognize and harmonize the many different aspects of your life, you are on the path to health.

This comprehensive perspective is an essential element of sustainable individual and communal health, and the foundation on which deep medicine is based.

Aspects of Healing

If health is about balance and healing is about change, then we could say that healing is the journey to the balance and wholeness of health. Growth, aging, sickness, recovery, and death are also processes of change. Healing is also forgiveness, confession, reconciliation, and rectification. In broadening the definition of healing, Jeanne Achterberg includes the following important aspects of healing in her book *Woman as Healer* (1990, p. 194):

1. Healing is a lifelong journey toward wholeness.

2. Healing is remembering what has been forgotten about connection, unity, and interdependence among all things, living and nonliving.

3. Healing is embracing what is most feared.

4. Healing is opening what has been closed, softening what has been hardened into obstruction.

5. Healing is entering into the transcendent, timeless moment when one experiences the divine.

6. Healing is creativity, passion, and love.

7. Healing is seeking and expressing self in its fullness, its light and shadow, its male and female.

8. Healing is learning to trust life.

Health does not mean being completely free of illness or defying death indefinitely. It is about human values as well as lab values. It is more than the absence of symptoms; it means a wholeness and alignment in living our lives—a dynamic and constantly changing balance that acknowledges the soundness of our physical state, the wholesomeness of our lifestyle, the values and virtues that define our behavior, our intimate and collective relationships, the meaning and purpose of our work in the world, and the cyclical and spiritual dimensions of our existence. It requires attention to our inner domains as well as to our outer world. It is not a static destination at which we will sometime arrive and then reside indefinitely. Daily, hourly, and even more frequent course corrections are the norm. How you feel at lunchtime is likely to have changed by dinnertime. You are a different person in the morning than the one who went to bed the previous night.

Thus, health may be seen as the dynamic manifestation of whatever you think, feel, say, do, and are, whereas healing may be seen as a change in anything that positively influences the delicate balance that is your health—from medications to relationships, from foods to thoughts, and from workplace to worship.

Ultimately, everything is either health creating or health negating. Everything!

The Four-Fold Way

Angeles Arrien, Ph.D., is a cultural anthropologist, healer, and educator whose work reveals how the wisdom of indigenous peoples is relevant to contemporary life. Her goal is to reunite us with our ecological and cultural roots. In her approach, she honors the health of the inner house of ourselves and the outer house of the world in which we live. Her inspiring book *The Four-Fold Way* (1993) is a transformative anthropological synthesis of timeless teachings relevant to modern times.

The Four-Fold Way teaches eight universal healing principles found in many cultures. Review the following list and assess for yourself where you are supporting your health and well-being and where you are not attending to these health care issues:

1. Balanced diet

2. Regular exercise

3. Time for play, fun, and laughter

4. Music, singing, chanting, and dancing

5. Love, touch, relationship, and support networks

6. Engaging in creative pursuits in work and leisure

7. Time spent in nature, with beauty, and in healing environments

8. Faith and belief in the sacred, spiritual, or unknowable

The principles and practices of *The Four-Fold Way* call us to choose to be fully present (that is, to show up in the moment); to pay attention (to listen to what has heart and meaning); to tell the truth without blame or judgment; and to be open to outcome rather than attached to it. Furthermore, *The Four-Fold Way* challenges us, in the spirit of honest, timely, direct communication, to say what is so (to tell the truth), to say what we mean (to operate with integrity), and to do what we say we will do (to build trust). These are elemental and universal health-creating principles and practices that foster character development, presence, and well-being.

WHAT IS ILLNESS? WHAT IS DISEASE?

Now that we understand what health and healing are, what is the difference between disease and illness, when both may be associated with life events, stress, and disconnections between our most deeply held values and dreams and our actual circumstances?

When I returned to San Francisco after the death of my father in Arizona, I hit a post in the hospital parking lot with my car, threw my back out stepping distractedly off a curb, and came down with a serious upper respiratory infection. Even without detailed identification of the specific cause-and-effect relationships involved—for instance, increased susceptibility to infection because of my immune system being suppressed by stress—my health-related responses are a compelling illustration of the associations between one's life circumstances and state of well-being.

"Disease" is considered an abnormality in the structure and function of bodily organs and systems, whereas "illness" includes all the difficulties that a disease creates: dependency, fear, isolation, loss, grief, inability to make a living, and limitations in the activities of daily life, such as eating, moving about, and personal hygiene. "Illness" might even include the experience of being devalued personally and socially during a sickness. While doctors may be primarily interested in the recognition and treatment of disease, patients are mainly concerned with the difficulties and discomforts that their sickness imparts—their illness. Each view is incomplete, and both are necessary for accessing the richly multilayered arenas of health and healing.

In his landmark book *Anatomy of an Illness* (1979), Norman Cousins wrote about being hospitalized for a progressive paralytic condition of the spine. He described his response to his disease and, in doing so, the distinctions between disease and illness. Cousins reported his feeling of helplessness; the fear of never being able to function normally again; his aversion to being thought of as a complainer; the desire not to add to his family's burden; his isolation and the conflict between the terror of loneliness and the desire to be left alone; and, most importantly, the longing for the warmth of human contact. During his hospitalization and care, he wished much more for a warm smile or an outstretched hand than for the offerings of modern medical science. However, he found that the latter were more readily available than the former.

Illness and its attendant suffering can occur even in the absence of a measurable disease. A large number of visits to the doctor are for complaints without an ascertainable pathologic basis. What's more, many episodes of being "sick" (colds, headaches, aches and pains, and minor injuries) are managed outside the formal health care system—

meaning that people are taking care of themselves as best they can, often without seeing a doctor.

Healing Lessons

In their classic 1978 article "Culture, Illness, and Care: Clinical Lessons from Anthropologic and Cross-Cultural Research," in the *Annals of Internal Medicine*, Arthur Kleinman, MD, and associates report a small but instructive study with relevant recommendations on distinguishing between disease and illness. Dr. Kleinman conducted the study in Taiwan using one hundred patients who visited indigenous healers. The majority were found to be suffering from disorders that fell into one of three main groups: self-limited diseases that resolved; chronic diseases that weren't life threatening, in which related psychological and social problems were the chief concerns; and somatization, in which physical complaints represented mental illness. (Mind and body are not separated in the Chinese medical construct, and mental illness has been somewhat culturally stigmatized.)

In a follow-up assessment, a small subgroup of ten of twelve patients reported their treatment as successful, even though not all physical symptoms had improved. The two patients who reported their treatment as unsuccessful were the only ones with severe medical or psychiatric disease (acute kidney infection and acute depression). The researchers interpreted their findings to mean that illness, not disease, predominates for most patients visiting indigenous healers. Treatment was considered successful when it impacted the patients' illness. The patients with documented pathologic diseases were not successfully treated by the indigenous healers.

To get at the distinction between disease and illness and to serve the large number of people seeking healing from their illness—not just a cure for a disease—Kleinman (1981, p. 106) has suggested the following open-ended questions as part of the doctor-patient conversation. You can also use them for your own personal assessment of the conditions and situations for which you do and don't seek professional health care:

1. What do you call your problem? What name does it have?

2. What do you think has caused your problem?

3. Why do you think it started when it did?

4. What does your sickness do to you? How does it work?

5. How severe is it? Will it have a short or long course?

6. What do you fear most about your sickness?

7. What are the chief problems your sickness has caused for you?

8. What kind of treatment do you think you should receive? What are the most important results you hope to receive from the treatment?

Engaging these questions personalizes your ailment, rather than objectifying it and holding it at arm's length. These questions are a way of bringing the objective, scientific world of medicine and health care into conversation with the subjective, social world in terms of your health and illness. They are a useful bridge to healing and part of a holistic approach to well-being. (You will learn more about bridging the inner and outer worlds as a path to wholeness and healing in chapter 7.)

THE CHARACTER OF HEALTH: SELF-ASSESSMENT

Anthropologic, cultural, emotional, and spiritual perspectives about health and healing move you beyond the pure science of symptoms, be they mental or physical, toward core issues such as fear, connection, trust, awe, belief, and love. In exploring your health issues, you will find yourself dealing with the need for authenticity, honesty, and compassion—true character issues, which are fundamental to the development of optimal health. Character is the combination of qualities and features that, when seen together, make up the moral and ethical fabric of an individual or group. On your path to well-being, the choice of a particular program, modality, or practitioner may become less important than the authentic engagement of your own character development.

Building character demands your rapt attention to the present moment. You must be alert not to wallow in past disappointments or wounds. You cannot waste your precious energy worrying or fantasizing about what might or might not happen. If you dissipate your life force on the past or the future, you won't have the personal resources to fully engage the present. You must learn from the past, yet the present is where you reside, and where you choose to heal the past and create the future. Remember the lessons and learning of the past without being ensnared or stuck there. Plan and prepare carefully for the future without investing completely in what may or may not come to pass.

Underlying character development and the true pursuit of health is self-responsibility. Beginning with honest and frequent self-assessment, you will progress to self-discovery, self-knowledge, and, ultimately, self-efficacy in acting upon what you learn. Your self-assessment can begin with four questions suggested by Wyatt Webb in his book *It's Not About the Horse—It's About Overcoming Fear and Self-Doubt* (2002). These questions need to be asked whenever you feel lost, stuck, or uncertain, and they can be used anytime, anyplace, and about any subject to help you locate yourself and determine your next small, smart step in the process of creating health and reducing risks to your well-being. These questions are a way of taking your "vital signs":

1. What am I thinking?

2. What am I feeling?

3. What am I doing?

4. How is it working?

If you can honestly say that things seem to be working well for you, then by all means continue along your present route. But if not, it's time to try something else or get some help. For example, if you're thinking about how uninspired you are at work or are feeling depressed, burned-out, and unable to make a move, it's clear that things aren't working. Something must be done to break the logjam. No matter how small the next step may seem—whether looking for job opportunities on the Internet, signing up for a class that sounds appealing, or making an appointment with a valued healer, counselor, mentor, or friend—the step in and of itself will improve depression, relieve anxiety, and set the wheels of change in motion.

Deep Medicine will help you determine the key questions that will catalyze the internal or external conversations most necessary for your health and healing. What might you ask that would move your quest for health and healing to the next level? You might ask a question such as "What is my desired personal breakthrough at this time related to my health or self-care?" Or you might ask questions to probe what is stopping you: "What's keeping me from doing what I really want to do? What resources do I possess right now that can support the change I desire? What beliefs or behaviors am I enslaved to that are holding me back?"

These questions are deeper than queries about carbohydrates or proteins, yoga or Spinning classes. They demand an in-depth appreciation of who you are, where you've come from, and where you're going. They are questions that plumb your purpose, your passion, your will, and your dreams. They are the questions that bring meaning and joy to your life—questions that you must determine for yourself and answer for yourself, not just once, but many times during the phases of healing and over the span of your life.

This approach to self-assessment, self-discovery, self-knowledge, and self-efficacy is deep work. It embodies the challenge of initiating and sustaining change. It is about attitude, attention, action, and the character to stick to a chosen course toward your desired goal. From this point forward, *Deep Medicine* will engage you in the development of your own personal program of change toward greater well-being.

QUICK FIX OR LASTING SOLUTION?

Compliance with and adherence to any medical or health program can be challenging to maintain. We are all seduced by the possibility of a short, sweet resolution to our challenges. There's nothing wrong with wanting solutions to be quick and easy—except that, in real life, this doesn't often occur. In exploring health issues, we inevitably find ourselves dealing with such necessities as penetrating self-inquiry; rigorous honesty about our strengths, weaknesses, resources, and obstacles; and ever-changing circumstances. In our quest for healing, we need commitment and discipline to sustain our course over time, a deep sense of responsibility to carry us toward our objectives, and the courage and humility to seek help where and when we need it.

An exercise program, a stress reduction course, the newest self-help book, or the latest diet, supplement, or vitamin may attract us with the promise of renewed health, but beware: Lost weight is gained back about 90 percent of the time; January's New Year's resolutions are often abandoned by March; the ten easy steps are either too easy and nothing happens or too hard and aren't done; and instant enlightenment isn't that fast, just as an "overnight success" is usually based on years of hard work. It's fairly safe to say that the quick fix or easy answer, as alluring as it might sound, is just plain illusory.

As you travel the path toward creating your own health and well-being, your character will be tested and you will be required to grow in the formation of that set of qualities referred to as your character. Character development is clearly an integral part of harnessing your healing power.

The path to healing is long, strewn with obstacles, and without end. Health is a moving target and the journey is not *to* it, but *about* it. It is about standing, walking, running, eating, resting, dancing, wishing, praying, thinking, feeling, learning, and choosing. The creation of health is a marathon, not a sprint, and it's never too early to begin. Don't wait for a crisis to jolt your awareness; the time to start on your road to healing is now. The trip can even be fun!

In the words of Martin Luther, "This life, therefore, is...not health but healing, not being but becoming, not rest but exercise; we are not what we shall be, but we are growing toward it; the process is not yet finished, but it is going on; this is not the end, but it is the road" (Luther, Jacobs, and Spaeth 1930, p. 31).

Deep Medicine proposes a process of lifelong learning and ongoing change—at your own pace, not as a time-constrained short course. This is foundation work, not a fresh coat of paint. No one teacher, no one philosophy or approach can provide all the answers. Each of us must create healing for ourselves, and success in this endeavor requires the development of true character.

Your energy belongs in the present, as has been espoused in the wisdom of many ages and traditions teaching us to be awake, mindful, ready, and in the now. The essence of your growth in life is to be present and to build your character. If you can do these two things, contentment and well-being will follow. The work of creating health and healing requires that you be present to win!

EXERCISES FOR CHAPTER 1: ASKING THE RIGHT QUESTIONS

Personal Health Assessment Questionnaire

Health and healing are a matter of bringing awareness to life. In order to do that, you have to assess your state of health—mental, emotional, physical, and spiritual—on an ongoing basis. Consider using a notebook or journal for the exercises that end each chapter. In doing so, you will write your own guidebook about the discoveries you make as to what works and what doesn't on your path to well-being.

The following questions, which are grouped in five general areas, should bring you in touch with many lifestyle issues. While your inherited genetics and the intangibles of luck, fate, and destiny play a large part in health, lifestyle is also a critical determinant of well-being—and you can actually do something about that! (These questions are adapted from an assessment tool owned by the Institute for Health and Healing at California Pacific Medical Center, San Francisco, California, and are used with permission.)

1. Overview

What breakthrough or change would you most like to achieve with regard to your health? How important is this change to you? How confident are you that you can achieve this change? Use a scale of your choosing (for instance, −10 to +10, or 1 to 10) to record the present level of the importance of this change, and then use the same scale to assess your confidence that you can do something about it. Consider your rankings and why they are at their current levels and not higher or lower.

What are your current and previous medical problems? Specifically, what symptoms are you experiencing? Are there recurring themes—physical, mental, emotional, or spiritual?

Can you identify areas of weakness? What about areas of strength?

What medications, vitamins, or natural remedies (for instance, herbs) are you currently using?

Do you know why you're using them?

Are they helping?

Are you aware of their effects—both good and bad? Have you monitored these effects with a symptom journal?

What significant illnesses run in your family? Are there any recurrent themes? Are you like your parents? Do you see your parents in your own illnesses? Review your family of origin, your parents and siblings, and note any aspects that relate to your present health status.

2. Life Habits

What do your food and drink say about you? Examine your diet for a typical week, including number of meals per day and how often you eat meat, dairy products, fish, vegetables, whole grains, and sweets. Are you satisfied with your present nutritional state?

Are you aware of why, what, where, when, and how you eat?

What are your addictions (tobacco, caffeine, alcohol, and so on), and why do you think you have chosen them?

What foods do you crave? When do you crave them? How do you respond to your craving?

What do you currently do for physical activity? What keeps you from exercising or engaging in physical activity? What encourages you to exercise or engage in physical activity? Are you satisfied with your present level of physical activity?

3. Work and Social History

What have been the most significant events in your life? How do you think they've impacted your health—both past and present?

What is your current job? Are you satisfied with it?

How does your job impact your health?

Would changing your job benefit your health?

Describe the relationship between work, play, and rest in your life. Is it a satisfactory ratio?

Where are you currently living? Are you satisfied with your environment?

What is your marital or living status? Are you satisfied with it?

Do you have social support networks to help you in times of distress? To share joyful times?

4. Body Image and Sexuality

Does your physical self-image encourage or discourage healthy behavior?

Are there issues in regard to your sexuality that affect your well-being?

5. Guiding Values

What values or principles guide you?

Do you have sayings you live by? (Common examples include "Keep a stiff upper lip," "Big boys don't cry," or "Be a good girl.")

How would you describe your spirituality? How important is it to you? Are you satisfied with the spiritual aspects of your life?

Do you pray? For yourself? For others?

Do you think your relationship with a higher power has anything to do with the quality of your life and health?

What is your understanding of the "greater good"?

What is your purpose?

What gives meaning to your life?

Do you have a concept of your life's dream?

How do you understand the concept of your fate, or destiny?

6. Summary

Having reviewed these various aspects of your life, how satisfied are you with the state of your health?

Given this assessment, can you identify insights and learnings about yourself that will impact your health plan?

Can you identify and prioritize changes that would serve your health?

Do you appreciate the difference between a "cure" for a disease or ailment and the larger concept of healing, which can occur even in the presence of an incurable disease?

Fast Track Self-Assessment

If the comprehensive health assessment above appears too complicated or too time-consuming, you can do a fast-track self-assessment by asking yourself these four key questions:

1. What am I thinking?

2. What am I feeling?

3. What am I doing about it?

4. How is it working for me?

CHAPTER 2

The Challenge of Change

It is not the strongest of the species that survives, nor the most intelligent, but the one most responsive to change.

—Charles Darwin

Not choice, but habit rules the unreflecting herd.

—William Wordsworth

Alone in his hospital room, his body ravaged with complications of alcoholism, Bill Wilson was filled with despair. He realized that what he had been, he could no longer be. He said later, as quoted by psychiatrist Mitchell Liester, "Lying there in conflict, I dropped into black depression. Momentarily, my prideful obstinacy was crushed. I cried out, 'Now I am ready to do anything!'" (1996, 14).

His world overturned, Wilson went on to recover and, together with Dr. Bob Smith, he founded Alcoholics Anonymous, supporting others through obstacle-strewn paths by helping them learn to make health-creating choices.

A heart attack, cancer diagnosis, death in the family, or failed job or relationship is often the crisis wake-up call that first announces how far a person's life has swung out of balance. The desire or willingness to make a change may occur when the discomfort, pain, or "dis-ease" of staying the same becomes greater than the resistance to and fear of change.

To be able to make choices and changes that are health creating and sustainable, you must understand and appreciate the influence that lifestyle choices have on your well-being and your capacity to heal. Each of us brings to the table the genetic hand we are dealt. Each of us also lives in an environment, whether pristine or toxic. And we all have varying degrees of access to medical care and healthful options. All of these components are critical to well-being, and you may not have much control over these factors. But one factor you do have significant control over—lifestyle choices—is responsible for a major proportion of the health equation.

What does it take to motivate a change in habits? Does a person have to hit bottom like Bill Wilson? What moves us to carry on or to throw in the towel? How much is enough? Where do we go from here? These questions lack precise answers because they stir the gut, touch the heart, and challenge the mind. And they are as relevant to the nature of being human as they are to the specifics of the issues that impact health.

CYCLES OF CHANGE

The theme of this chapter is the challenge of change. Even though humans are built for overall stability, we are changing from moment to moment. The person who makes a decision on Friday night to take off a bit of excess holiday weight is not the same person who wakes up Saturday morning and must stay on that program. Your thoughts, emotions, and physical body are in constant flux. You think differently if you are hungry, tired, afraid, bored, or under stress. Your emotions vary under the influences of internal hormones, the weather, where you are, who you are with, and what you're doing. Physiologically, you are undergoing constant cycles of breakdown and repair.

The neuroscience of learning, habit, and addiction has demonstrated that changing a habitual behavior requires much more conscious brain activity than acting in usual ways, on automatic pilot. This is why it really is harder to teach an old dog new tricks; it is still possible, just harder. Successful change requires not just a certain cookbook or running shoes, but the commitment, honest self-assessment, discipline, and flexibility to carry out the program you've chosen. Yet it is more than just choosing a program, and it's more than willpower alone or stubbornness. Everything you think, feel, say, and do—everything you are—is required to create, sustain, or recover a healthy life because, as you'll recall from chapter 1, health is literally about balance.

Living in balance is an elusive endeavor, and it's much easier said than done. Often you will be slightly off balance and in the process of making corrections to establish equilibrium somewhere in the middle, between extremes. You actually seek this alignment both consciously and unconsciously with frequent, subtle corrections; it's not unlike adjusting your steering and speed while driving a car, riding a bike, or walking along a crowded sidewalk or irregular path. Along the way, you have to make sharp turns and quick stops, and sometimes even back up. Internal and external phenomena can knock you off balance; therefore, you must constantly be aware of where your balance needle is pointing and make the necessary adjustments to remain upright and on your true course.

STRESS: TORTURE OR TEACHER?

Stress can disrupt your balance and lead you toward a breakdown (destructive, unhealthful change) or toward a breakthrough (constructive, healthful change). When you become ill, it is because of being stressed in some way, whether physical, mental, emotional, spiritual, or a combination of multiple sources. In the medical sense, *stress* is a cascade of internal, physiological responses to a threat. From an evolutionary standpoint, threats have generally been physical (such as dangerous encounters). These days, stress is more likely to be psychological (for example, worry). Whether the threat is real or imagined, short-term or long-term, it is mediated by similar physiologic phenomena. In general terms, these bodily reactions result in increased mental alertness, heart rate, blood pressure, muscle tension, and blood sugar levels and in decreased activity of the gastrointestinal (digestive) and immune systems.

Symptoms of stress involve all bodily systems in a broad range of manifestations, but in reality they are an expression of the body's wisdom. Our bodies were built for short bursts of intense activity, such as fleeing from a predator. The stress response is usually described as preparing us for fight or flight, but it can also result in a reaction of freezing. In women, stress can also stimulate a nurturing or nesting response. When physiologic stress responses are chronically activated, they become unsustainable and the symptoms of stress appear. When activated repeatedly by fears generated by memory or expectation, actions that can save us in a brief moment of crisis become health negating rather than health creating. Depending on the person and the circumstance, stress-related symptoms range from clarity to panic, anxiety to depression, hyperactivity to collapse, overeating to loss of appetite, crying to rage. Stress-related illness may appear as weight gain or weight loss, diarrhea or constipation, chest pain, irregular heartbeat, shortness of breath, or dizziness. Mental illness, cardiac disease, stomach and intestinal disorders, headache, back pain, skin problems, and autoimmune diseases such as chronic fatigue syndrome and fibromyalgia are just some of the conditions associated with stress.

Even though everyone has unique causes leading to imbalances, symptoms, and diseases—even where there are common agents operating, such as infections (bacteria, viruses)—stress shows where you need to change in order to feel better. For example, physical stress may be caused by too much work, not enough sleep, or exposure to a large dose of an infectious agent. Mental or emotional stress may come from excessive worry about what might happen or failure to let go of debilitating memories of what has happened. Spiritual stressors include lack of meaning or purpose in one's life, a disconnect between one's dreams or yearnings and one's circumstances, or an absence of faith or belief where faith or belief is desired.

Think about your life: Can you identify specific aspects where stress is affecting your well-being in negative or positive ways?

STRESS AS A GUIDE

Recognizing and managing stress can be a great source of guidance if you're aware of your body's messages. You'll notice that many stressors aren't necessarily bad things, just stress-evoking happenings. Illness and injury are certainly stressors, as are birth and death and most of life's milestones and crises. Work, whether too much or lack of, is a stressor. Relationships—romance, rejection, marriage, pregnancy, child rearing, divorce, death in the family, and so on—are stressors. A major decision, accident, natural disaster, decreased income, and even a big raise or windfall are also stressors.

Even if stress isn't an obvious contributor to the onset of a disease, stress management often becomes a relevant aspect of recovery in a comprehensive treatment plan. The more aware you are of the messages—the early warnings and symptoms your body is sending about how you're doing—the greater your opportunity to prevent a crisis or serious breakdown. Thus, the early recognition of weariness before it becomes complete fatigue, of subtle anxiety before it becomes a panic attack, of irritability before it becomes an angry outburst, or of a heart palpitation or twinge of pain before it becomes a heart attack can lead you to track the sources of stress, to modify the external causes as much as possible, and to set out to rebalance your internal homeostasis, or stability. The power of prevention and early detection is why, when you embark on a wilderness adventure, your guide will caution you to drink before you're thirsty, eat before you're hungry, and rest before you're tired. An ounce of prevention really can be worth more than a pound of cure.

This is how stress becomes a teacher and a healer—when you can hear the messages and are willing to act on the guidance before a breakdown occurs. As an exercise, track some situations that cause you to feel stressed or overwhelmed. Are you aware of any early warning signals that could alert you and allow you to prevent or limit the risk of a full-blown meltdown? Recognition of these early warning signals is part of accessing your sources of healing power.

Managing stress is an arena that brings you face-to-face with the challenge not simply of reducing symptoms, but of changing your ways. These changes usually involve not only the circumstances of your external world, but awareness of what you're experiencing in your inner world as well. This is where the potential for breakdown becomes the possibility for breakthrough.

A PERSONAL SYSTEM FOR CHANGE

Finding programs to manage stress or enhance well-being and healing isn't really the difficult part. We often know what we need to do or have access to those who can guide us regarding what to do.

The difficulty, it appears, is in actually doing it.

So, what prevents anyone from doing the things needed to make health-creating changes? Why do people not do what it takes to manage an illness optimally, whether taking medicines as prescribed, resting as recommended, quitting smoking, becoming physically active, eating right, or managing stress? What are you presently doing or not doing that you know could improve your state of well-being?

That which cries out for healing in each person is as unique as that individual's genetic makeup, history, and present circumstances. Although it usually takes a crisis to bring the state of our health to our attention, wouldn't it be wonderful to begin to make health-creating choices and changes *before* a crisis occurs? Learning to walk on a balance beam is easier when it's on the ground than when it's suspended several feet in the air. Establishing a solid foundation for health before a major crisis can help you cope—and may even prevent serious health issues from developing.

To start a shift toward creating a personal health-generating plan, you need to be your own teacher in your private school of self-knowledge—and to complete your homework. The curriculum involves educating yourself about what health is as it relates to lifestyle choices, then learning about yourself—your own lifestyle habits, beliefs, and choices—and developing the skills needed for change. Coursework includes character development (see chapter 1), honest self-exploration, connecting with your life dreams, achieving core competencies, facing fears, and accurately naming your problems and goals. To put it in medical terms, this is a process of making your "diagnosis" and defining your treatment plan.

As you search for the next right plan to move you toward a desired change, it's valuable to remember that the programs that actually work the best are those you devise for yourself. It is your dance, and insofar as you choreograph your own steps rather than following a routine devised by someone else, you will find your dance more meaningful and evocative. When this dance expresses your deepest concerns and needs, the performance will be stunning and compelling to you and to those who witness it.

This is deep medicine.

THE POWER OF LIFESTYLE CHOICES AND CHANGES

Your lifestyle choices are literally a matter of life and death. A 2008 article in the *New England Journal of Medicine* reported that "preventable causes of death, such as tobacco smoking, poor diet and physical inactivity, and misuse of alcohol have been estimated to be responsible for 900,000 deaths annually—nearly 40 percent of total yearly mortality in the United States" (Cohen, Neumann, and Weinstein 2008, p. 661).

This means that in the United States, four in ten deaths from significant illness annually are related to lifestyle choices that are within each person's power to recognize and control. Data show that lifestyle changes involving diet, exercise, stress management, and social connections improve physical well-being and reduce the death rate across all categories. In other words, any and all constructive lifestyle changes that you make are health-creating choices.

The very nature of real change often demands that you break behavior patterns or habits that, although detrimental to your health and well-being, feel safe, are known, and provide a sense of stability. Thus, truly meaningful change requires leaving your comfort zone. Habits and stable patterns of behavior are necessary; otherwise we would live in chaos. This makes it difficult to leave one's established patterns of behavior even when they are no longer useful or health creating. Here, again, we encounter the need for balance. Although it is necessary to choose to leave one's comfort zone, this action requires discernment. Seeking a "stretch goal," something commonly sought in the workplace, can be a stimulating experience. However, reaching too far can create fear, worry, and stress, all of which can undermine the potential for success. As you go about choosing and changing, you must make adjustments that are small enough that you don't completely lose your balance, yet take steps large enough that you do make progress.

THE STAGES OF CHANGE

A well-known Zen master visits New York City. Experiencing all the city has to offer, he goes up to a hot dog vendor and says, "Make me one with everything." The hot dog vendor fixes a link and hands it to the Zen master, who pays with a twenty dollar bill. The vendor puts the bill in the cash box and closes it. After a few moments of waiting patiently, the Zen master asks, "Where's my change?" The vendor responds, "Change must come from within."

Each of us has recurrent patterns of stuck behavior—habitual responses that repetitively lead us to dead-end relationships, frustrating work situations, chronic unhappiness, unfulfilled yearnings, or illness. Changing these patterns is often more like major surgery than a quick adjustment. It requires insight, courage, and hard work. Only deep, fundamental internal change sustains meaningful and lasting external growth and progress. Even in a collective context, lasting social change often requires deep personal transformation.

Change, and our potential to change, is a process that often is described as occurring in the following stages (Prochaska, Norcross, and DiClemente 1994):

1. **Precontemplation equilibrium:** You are not yet interested in changing, or aware of the need for change.

2. **Contemplation or disorientation:** You get the first inklings that a change might be in order, from internal or external sources.

3. **Preparation or exploration:** You begin to think about, talk about, and research options.

4. **Action or reorientation:** You begin to take active steps to change your ways.

5. **New equilibrium or maintenance:** You continue to practice what you've learned and to create a new homeostasis, or balance.

THE FOUR CORE COMPETENCIES

So often, people have turned their health over to the "experts" rather than appreciating their own power to catalyze and sustain lasting change. In our culture, staying healthy has been equated with periodically going to the doctor, rather than fostering healthful ways of living on a daily basis. To overcome the inertia and begin to make health-creating changes, you must look beyond the external symptoms of your imbalances and inquire within. Here you will not use just your rational, objective mind; you will be required to engage your imagination, trust your instincts and intuition, and focus your attention on well-defined intentions for health-creating action.

Change cannot simply be prescribed or imposed from the outside. Each individual decides for himself or herself where he is, where he is going, what she has to deal with, and how and when she will do so. The path and timeline through the stages vary from person to person, and progress occurs only as readiness for the next stage appears. Sometimes there is a seemingly backward movement, a long pause, or a relapse, a situation that requires assessment and tracking of what happened and restarting the change process with appropriate course corrections—for example, avoiding people and places that foster the undesired behaviors, or surrounding oneself with a network of friends and family who are supportive of the desired goal.

For the sake of clarity and to create manageable parts, we can think of the stages of change as the application of a set of core competencies: investigation, inspiration, initiation, and integration. These competencies parallel the classical stages of change as described above:

- **Investigation** is gaining awareness and curiosity, as well as gathering information and being educated about knowledge bases, skill sets, and useful tools for change.

- **Inspiration** involves determining the importance of various changes and building motivation and confidence that what is desired can be accomplished.

- **Initiation** involves actively taking steps, such as deciding exactly what to do, defining a structure for change by planning when and how to do it, and then actually doing it, through behavior change.

- **Integration** involves incorporating new behaviors into daily activities through repeated practice, making necessary course corrections, learning the skill of self-negotiation and using it successfully and often, and finding support to help stay the course.

One reason I like to think in terms of the core competencies is that change isn't a process you go through once, and then you're done. It's a process you engage in again and again throughout your life.

Investigation

Investigation is the competency needed when the first inklings arise that change might be warranted. Perhaps friends tell you that you seem sad, remote, or distracted, or that you're drinking too much or not keeping commitments. Or maybe you realize that your clothes fit a bit too tightly, you're getting a bit winded walking up the slope of the driveway, or a lump is getting bigger, not going away.

Then you begin to think about, talk about, and explore possibilities. This is a time when you grow your awareness through frequent self-assessment, using the four key questions from chapter 1:

1. What am I thinking?

2. What am I feeling?

3. What am I doing?

4. How is it working?

During this time, your curiosity comes alive, and you seek more information from friends, the Internet, libraries, and others with similar problems. You appreciate that things are not quite right. You are building a data bank.

This competency correlates with the first three classic stages of change: precontemplation equilibrium, contemplation or disorientation, and preparation or exploration. In this period you observe, describe, identify, name, and carefully begin to track that which you intend to change. You must name accurately, for it is equivalent to making a diagnosis, and only through correct diagnosis will you devise the proper treatment.

Inspiration

The second core competency useful in navigating the process of creating health is finding inspiration. This competency correlates with the second and third classic stages of change: contemplation or disorientation and preparation or exploration. It is not enough to notice your faults, bad habits, and need for growth and change or have them pointed out. You must be motivated to do something about whatever it is you might want to change. While it is true that you can be influenced or inspired by peers or by people important to you, and by data and success stories, that kind of inspiration often is washed away by the perspiration of the hard work actually required to achieve your desired goal.

Ultimately, the inspiration to begin and the motivation to carry on must come from within. No amount of willpower, stubbornness, or determination will be enough if you aren't driven by an inner source of motivation and yearning. When it comes right down to the basics, there are really only two things that motivate anyone to change: something that you really want (for example, good health, long life, meaningful work, lasting relationships, or a safe environment); and something that you really don't want (for example, to die prematurely, to live with the constant threat of violence, or to not be able to care for yourself or your loved ones).

Once you begin on a path of change, you will need to renew your motivation and inspiration again and again. Seeing the fruits of your labors is helpful here; results are a key source of motivation. Weight loss, improved results on lab tests, improved mood and higher energy levels, or a new job—all contribute to renewing your initial inspiration and supporting your motivation to keep on keeping on. You may also be moved by teachers, classes, partners, friends, and family members who support your goals and aid your progress.

Initiation

Initiation is the third core competency. It correlates with the fourth classic stage of change: action or reorientation. This is where you begin to take active steps to change your behavior, and where attention is critical. Bringing your attention to something literally turns on the brain, enhancing the possibility of learning something new and then, through repetition and practice, remembering it. Good and bad habits are formed as thoughts, feelings, and behaviors are repeated, stimulating development of new brain synapses and even adaptation and new growth of brain cells. At this time, you must also define boundaries for your creativity and aspirations. To do this you have to set priorities and make decisions and choices.

Everyone has a full gamut of aspirations. Some are lofty, some practical. Among the multitude of possible actions, some are loud and demanding, others more remote and perhaps more alluring. What to do? If you make choices that are consistent with your underlying philosophy or perspective, they will be health creating and life sustaining. You need a philosophy that braids scientific and spiritual legacies, that acknowledges your biology and your life story. This will bring you to insightful thinking, compassionate feeling, and service-oriented action. This will support a balanced daily existence, not necessarily free of difficult choices or conflict, but consistent with your personal vision.

The following questions can help guide your decision-making process as you set priorities, directions, and limits:

- Does the decision feel right?

- Does it seem rational?

- Is it consistent with my concept of truth?

- Is it in line with my integrity?

- Is it sustainable for my personal economy, for the environment, and for future generations?

If you hear a voice of doubt, even far in the distance, don't ignore it. Listen to it early in your decision-making process—it may be a fear you need to acknowledge, or it may be your own internal voice of wisdom, a source of healing power, that you are hearing.

How we begin something is critical to how the entire project will go. Start where you are, knowing with full confidence that small steps are the way to start. First steps should be not only small, but also simple, not too hard, and interesting. If your steps are the right size for you and pleasing in their results and the process of taking them, you will repeat them. This way they are actually accomplished, and without undue distress, setting the stage for the next appropriate small step. Taking on too much too soon leads to self-sabotage, whereas small steps, consistently done, lead to big changes. At this point, it's useful to enhance your success by bringing structure to your project in the form of good planning and sensible expectations, and by ensuring you have adequate support from family, friends, and others who will cheer you on and encourage you not to procrastinate.

Integration

Integration is the fourth core competency necessary for initiating and sustaining change. This competency corresponds to the fifth classic stage of change. In this phase, you establish and maintain a new equilibrium. You practice what you have learned and create a new homeostasis, or balance, for yourself. You continue to ingrain good habits as you repeat constructive behaviors that reward you with desired results, which become motivation for continued progress. Walking in nature, attending a yoga class, adhering to stress reduction practices, eating healthful foods, and seeking supportive groups become incorporated in your daily life. Even during the inevitable periods when progress slows and you plateau, these new behaviors persist because you value the results that you can track through your ongoing self-assessments. You continue to develop health-promoting character traits by telling yourself the truth and experiencing the joy that comes from aligning your inner desires and goals with your external reality.

NEGOTIATING FOR CHANGE

When your health-creating actions are coherent with your inner yearnings and life dreams, you have the greatest potential to sustain those actions over time. Being in touch and staying in touch with those things that reside in the realm of spirit and are beyond intellect and objective analysis, such as your perceived purpose, meaning, passion, and calling, will feed your process of change and be experienced as a sense of joy and contentment with your quest. To maintain this alignment with your physical, mental, emotional, and spiritual arenas requires ongoing negotiations with yourself as you face frequent and repeated decision points and the need for course corrections. For example, do you spend the afternoon on the couch or on your bicycle? Finish a project at work or attend your child's Little League game? Eat a bacon cheeseburger or a spinach salad? These and countless other health-related choices will appear many times every day. Being able to negotiate with yourself in a compassionate way will go a long way toward making your attempts at initiating and sustaining constructive change successful.

To accomplish these negotiations and make healthful choices, you need to know where you are, keep your desired goal in mind, and be able to recover and forgive yourself when you veer from your course. You will go off your diet, feel too tired to exercise, react with anger when you would have preferred patience, fall off the wagon, or act mean-spirited or selfish when generosity would have been the better choice. In these circumstances, you cannot be overly critical or judge yourself too harshly. Your self-talk must be fair and generous, neither inflating nor devaluing what is happening and how you are progressing. Doing this competently will keep you on course as well as get you back on track when you wander off your desired path. Often our self-talk can be hypercritical and excessively judgmental. You must learn to be a fair witness to yourself, neither inflating nor glossing over your strengths and weaknesses. Fair self-talk is essential for fruitful self-negotiation.

A SHIFT IN PERSPECTIVE

I never learned to stand on my head as a child.

I had often been challenged in my youth to stand on my own two feet or to sit or stand up straight like a big boy, or a man. But unlike most children, I never ventured onto my head upside down.

I'll never forget the day, as a grown man fifty years old, that I first succeeded in balancing myself upside down. It was a goal I was determined to achieve. It had taken years of meditation for mental equanimity and years of tai chi for fluidity and readiness for a serious yoga practice, then months of practice, instruction, guidance, coaching, and support to first get me comfortably, solidly upside down—beyond the fear and uncertainty.

What I discovered was a new perspective, a new confidence, and an enhanced sense of self-respect. As a mature man steeped in science, trusting of expertise, and impressed with excellence and success, I experienced my own balance and strength in a new way when completely turned over. Now as I stand on my head (or my hands) for longer periods, I am growing in balance, alignment, and ease. I feel a sense of accomplishment, and it's fun! I am resonating in a posture that has a wisdom of its own and gives me a whole new lens through which to view the world.

When you change your viewpoint, you see things differently. New possibilities arise that shift you beyond your usual ways of thinking, feeling, and acting. A sudden breakthrough may occur, or such a shift may occur slowly, after months of daily, subtle changes. Seeing things in a new way isn't about joining a cult or giving up beliefs; it's about connecting to internal wisdom, trusting your inner voice, and responding to its messages. This is one way true healing begins, through awakening your inner guiding wisdom.

Sometimes a transformative shift is necessary to get beyond obvious issues to underlying needs and the importance of changing certain patterns of behavior. Before behavior patterns can be changed, they must be seen and acknowledged, which can involve a host of dimensions: perspective, outlook, worldview, perception, and insight.

A familiar shift occurs in the Dickens classic *A Christmas Carol*, as Ebenezer Scrooge, visited by his ghosts, suddenly is able to see things from a totally different perspective and is radically transformed. Why was Scrooge moved to change? He was forced to recognize recurrent patterns in his life that were cruel—patterns that imprisoned rather than protected him. Do you recognize any such patterns in your life?

Dr. Elisabeth Targ, a psychiatrist and former research colleague at the Institute for Health and Healing, introduced me to the work of psychologists William R. Miller and Joseph C'deBaca. They studied individuals who reported sudden transformative change. The volunteer subjects reported having been "transformed and noting...a deep shift in core values, feelings, attitudes or actions" (1994, p. 259). Here are the top four shifts in valued priorities reported by men and women as a result of their sudden transformative experience:

Men's Priority Shifts		Women's Priority Shifts	
Before	*After*	*Before*	*After*
Wealth	Spirituality	Family	Growth
Adventure	Personal peace	Independence	Self-esteem
Achievement	Family	Career	Spirituality
Pleasure	God's will	Fitting in	Happiness

CHANGE TALK

Motivation and confidence are key predictors of a person's readiness to change. You must appreciate the importance of making a change and have reasonable confidence that you can succeed. If these two qualities are lacking, your chances of successfully changing are small.

You can be guided by the advice of experts, but part of the true pursuit of health entails accepting personal responsibility. Finding your own path requires appreciation of the multidimensional existence in which you live. It also requires identifying what matters and building the confidence and the courage to act on what you discover. As you read *Deep Medicine* and do the exercises at the end of each chapter, you will begin to define this path for yourself. However, taking responsibility for playing an active role in your own health and healing is not the same as blaming or judging failed modalities or yourself in relation to them. The important point is to give your chosen course your best shot by working in collaboration with your health care team, and then be open to the outcome.

In their superb book *Motivational Interviewing* (2002), William Miller and fellow psychologist Stephen Rollnick emphasize the importance of motivation being evoked rather than prescribed. For example, physicians are taught to diagnose illnesses and prescribe treatment. Compliance with prescribed treatment regimens, however, is often dismal. It is well-known that most people don't take medicines as prescribed, comply with treatment instructions, stick to prescribed diets, and so on. Even when they do succeed initially, they often backslide (regaining lost weight or discontinuing an exercise program, for example) as the initial inspiration is diluted by the hard work required to sustain the desired change. What motivates a person to begin a program of change may not provide sufficient motivation to continue such a program.

Miller and Rollnick describe "change talk" as one of the simplest and best parameters to observe in ascertaining someone's readiness to change. If suggestions for change are met with resistance talk ("That's a good idea, but..."; "I know that, however..."; "I've tried that and it didn't help..."), it's a strong indicator that the person isn't ready to take action and change. In these circumstances, more preparation is necessary to evoke an internal desire and motivation to change. When, on the other hand, change talk occurs ("Yes, I'm ready at last"; "I can't take it anymore"; "It's time to do something about this and stop just talking or thinking about it"), it's a good sign that the time is ripe for change.

These distinctions may seem obvious and simplistic. Nevertheless, they are some of the best indicators for predicting the potential for change, both for yourself and for others.

SUSTAINABLE CHANGE

Clearly, preparation and planning for change must be realistic, and initial steps must be few and small enough to allow early success.

You need to fortify yourself for the long haul, not for a quick fix, and your motivation to change must come from within, not be imposed upon you or prescribed by external sources. Your inner wisdom must be tapped and your inner sources of healing power awakened and harnessed.

Sustainable change can occur in as little as three to six weeks if you are in a state of awareness and readiness. The implication in this twenty-one- to forty-two-day interval is that if you practice a new behavior daily for this period of time, the new behavior will be habituated. That said, it's difficult to pinpoint a time frame with absolute precision; what's important to take away is that you must begin practicing the new behavior for any change to occur at all. What is true is that incorporation of new behavior into one's living patterns is dose related. That is, the more often you practice a behavior, the more likely it will be integrated and persist. A little bit each day is a useful approach.

Is the reverse true? That if you don't do a behavior for twenty-one to forty-two days it will permanently disappear? Possibly, but it is much less likely. It may be true for sucking your thumb; however, addictions such as alcoholism or smoking tobacco aren't likely to disappear that easily. In fact, the wounds of the toughest addictions leave residue akin to scars in the pathways of our brains, and old behaviors may resurface unexpectedly. Therefore, constant vigilance is required to prevent relapse or the resurgence of destructive behavior patterns.

Because eliminating a destructive habit is more difficult than establishing a new constructive habit, learning new, constructive behaviors as a way to displace destructive behaviors is an ancient approach to the management of "bad" habits. The practice of yoga, for example, provides healthful practices such as postures, breathing, and relaxation, which quiet the mind, strengthen the body, and expand the spirit to foster the development of constructive behaviors and displace self-defeating, nonproductive habits.

Small changes can be a useful way to start. If you don't bring home any ice cream, for instance, it will be easier not to eat it when you get a craving. If you can break your behavior patterns into small enough fragments, decisions about what to do may become easier.

Rather than planning a major workout and never getting out of your chair because the task seems too big, just decide to get up when the thought first hits you that you need some exercise. Then get yourself into your workout clothes, then out the door—even if you haven't decided exactly what form of exercise you'll do or where you'll go. A ten-minute walk done once, twice, or even three times a day is better than a two-hour trip to the gym that never happens.

THE FEAR OF CHANGE AND THE COURAGE TO CHANGE

From an evolutionary perspective, fear has contributed to both fostering and limiting change, and to preserving the species. We are programmed to be afraid. It is a survival need, as is stability, which is another force of nature that can limit the capacity to change. Stable patterns are necessary lest we live in chaos; however, they make it difficult to abandon entrenched behaviors, even those that are no longer useful, constructive, or health creating. And fear can keep you from changing when you don't want to risk a step into unknown territory; for example, some people choose not to leave an unfulfilling job or an abusive relationship because they fear the unknown more than the known. On the other hand, fear can also motivate change in order to avoid something you're afraid of, such as dying young—as one of your parents might have.

The very nature of real change demands that you break behavior patterns or habits that—while they may be detrimental to your health and well-being—feel safe, are known, and provide a sense of stability. Though we may profess to welcome new possibilities, meaningful change means leaving one's safety zone. Courage is thus required for change, because sometimes your personal truth may be counter to that of a peer group or accepted convention or your own image of yourself. Courage doesn't imply being free of fear or uncertainty. Rather, it means acting constructively in the presence of fear. Courage comes in living your own authentic life and coming in contact with your own gifts and talents, passions, calling, meaning, purpose, and life dreams.

Being yourself may mean standing up for something unpopular or moving forward with action that is unfamiliar and challenging.

When you are in fear, creative possibilities are constricted. Can you think of any fears that stand in the way of your well-being at this time? How do you go about facing your fears, whether real or imagined?

You can begin to transform your fear by being fully present. This reduces fears conjured up by memories and minimizes your worry about what might happen, which is what fuels most fears. When you're deeply engaged in what's happening now, it's less likely that you will be immobilized with fear—even if you actually are in a physically dangerous situation.

The challenge of change lies in being discerning about what you fear. This is where your capacity to choose your thoughts can either support your goal to be less fearful or propel you toward a life of perpetual anxiousness and worry. By choosing health-creating thoughts, you can build trust through the expression of appreciation, acknowledgment, respect, and understanding, thus reducing fear-based behaviors. As you practice such aspects of love as gratitude, forgiveness, and acceptance, your need to be in control will lessen and you will appreciate what you attract into your life.

Over time, the practice of being fully present in what is happening now—often referred to as mindfulness—can help reduce fear. It begins with bringing your attention to and being completely absorbed in what is happening in the present moment. From this place of attentiveness, the source of a fear can be tracked by listening to the messages your body is delivering and by noticing where those messages are coming from.

For example, where is the tension, the pain? Are you having difficulty breathing? Are you anxious? About what? This examination requires your quiet, undivided attention. You can begin the practice of being quietly present and tracking your bodily responses, thoughts, and feelings with the deep minute and the four practices explained in chapter 4. Many meditation, contemplation, and affirmation practices can facilitate your skill at this tracking by teaching you to not lose your concentration or awareness because of distractions such as noise. With time and practice, these approaches can circumvent fear. In the meantime, you might like to try this simple technique: When you find yourself afraid, say your name three times, breathe into the bodily site of the fear, acknowledge that "I am afraid," and affirm, "I can do what needs to be done."

HAPPINESS: ACCENTUATE THE POSITIVE

Reducing stress and reducing fear are aspects of the pursuit of health. What of building on the positive and increasing happiness? Often people are seduced by the medical model of eliminating the negative—that is, taking care of the disease. Rather than trying to reject something you don't want, such as fear, you can accentuate the positive, build on your strengths, and grow something that you *do* want, such as happiness. In their book *What Happy People Know* (2002), Dan Baker, Ph.D., and Cameron Stauth describe qualities of happiness, tools for developing it, and traps that can undermine true happiness. Happiness—a feeling of joy, contentment, or delight—is a desired state for most people. However, we can confuse intensity, adventure, and pleasure seeking with joy, contentment, and delight.

What is it that makes you happy—truly happy? Where do you find your happiness: at work, at home, out in nature, alone, with others?

People may look for happiness—as we do for love—in the wrong places. The qualities of happiness include being loved and loving; having a sense of freedom that allows the capacity to make choices; being proactive, or acting rather than reacting; seeing life in a context greater than oneself and appreciating the big picture, the greater good, and a higher power; and, of course, enjoying the security of health. We have been warned that we can't buy, will, demand, or mandate happiness, and in truth, once your most basic material needs have been met, it's unlikely that you'll find increased happiness through the external search for the perfect job, mate, home, or adventure. Neither major triumphs (for example, winning the lottery) nor catastrophes (health crises or natural disasters) seem to result in sustained, long-term (beyond a year) changes in the level of one's happiness.

True happiness seems to be more related to your state of mind than to your circumstances or the impact of transitory, external events. Because happiness is so directly related to your inner landscape, you can impact your level of happiness by your thoughts, emotions, and actions. One implication of this is that what you let into your sacred interior by what you watch, listen to, and talk about has an impact on your mood and level of happiness. Your food for thought must be as clean and health creating as the food you eat. That is why it's so important to do such things as read the classics and the wisdom and sacred literature from around the world, find some daily quiet time for reflection, and count your blessings and share them with others through acts of service and kindness. You must fill yourself with the observations and advice of sages, seers, and elders, not sound bites, hype, and advertising. At the same time, you must limit your exposure to calamity-oriented, sensationalistic news, comparing your situation to others, and desiring more. Everything you want for your own happiness needs to be seen in the context of its impact, cost, and consequences in the big picture and in relationship to the greater good, not just for its isolated impact on you.

You can literally practice building your happiness level in these ways and learn to be happy. As you find direction through quiet introspection and constructive contribution, and as you are appreciated and respected for who you really are, happiness will find you. Happiness comes from feeling good (health), doing good (compassionate service), and being good (building awareness, character, values, and meaningful purpose). Growth in happiness will also lead to or be associated with growth in self-worth. Action that serves your state of mind, bringing you toward equanimity and contentment with regard to your inner landscape, will also change your appreciation of the external circumstances of your life, causing you to see them differently. The reverse is not true, however; that is, changing your external circumstances without doing the inner work won't have the same impact on your inner landscape or your self-worth.

As you see yourself as more worthy, you'll be able to give and receive with greater ease. Being happy, fearless, curious, flexible, resourceful, and openhearted are all character traits that contribute to reducing fear, stress, and a sense of being overwhelmed—prime sources of health-negating behaviors and choices, and prime limiters of desired change. The development of these positive character traits is deep medicine, because it is character that empowers you to confront and overcome obstacles to the successful completion of your desired health-creating changes.

SUMMER WAKE-UP

As a healer, I know that it is necessary to diagnose impeccably and honestly. Yet sometimes it is very difficult to see ourselves clearly. It is quite interesting that we can see ourselves only in a mirror or as we are reflected back to ourselves by others. Smiles, hugs, and nodding are welcome reflections, while turning away, grimacing, and argument are ways we would rather not be reflected back.

Not long ago, my wife, Susy, and I arrived in British Columbia, Canada, for our annual summer vacation. We arrived tired, as usual, after the long drive from San Francisco and the multiple ferry crossings to reach our sylvan island destination.

The year had been rewarding, stimulating, and meaningful, with full schedules of work, travel, and family and social get-togethers. I didn't feel burned-out or stressed-out, just ready for summer vacation—a ritual I have loved since childhood and the countdown until school was out. I work hard, but I also ensure downtime, practice yoga regularly, walk daily, exercise vigorously at least one day each weekend, and try to practice what I preach. I was ready for a vacation, but not prepared for what followed: The bottom fell out!

I slept ten to twelve hours each night and looked forward to my afternoon nap. Vertical activities such as hiking and biking were fine in short bursts and as long as they didn't interfere with my horizontal needs for sleep, naps, and rest. My belly responded with an untwisting complete with gurgling, cramps, and loss of appetite. My dreams, both day and night, were vivid, imaginative, and full of possible explanations for my symptoms—most of them dark and distressing.

After several days of rest, my sleep modulated. My recovery wasn't as rapid as my collapse, and I was determined to see beyond my symptoms even as they improved. Obviously, I had been exhausted but failed to recognize or admit it. How had I been so oblivious to my own situation? I had clearly ignored or denied visceral messages about my state of well-being. "What's the message in this experience? What's the meaning?" I asked myself.

Even as an astute, knowledgeable doctor trained to see symptoms and warning signs in others and to name things accurately, I had blind spots in my inner vision and ability to see myself. My inner listening and ability to hear myself were dulled, deficient, and reduced. I hadn't been fully present with myself. I hadn't named my signs or symptoms or diagnosed myself well, and so I couldn't take care of myself well.

During my summer holiday time, I gave in to the reality of my state. My task was to heal—something I recommended to others regularly and now medicine that I had to take myself. And it certainly wasn't bitter medicine: I paid great attention to getting enough rest. I ate consciously and well. I practiced yoga, starting with relaxing, restorative poses. I had frequent massages, meditated regularly, and exercised daily. I spent plenty of time outside in nature and with family and friends. After my restful vacation, I didn't want to go back to my oblivious state or ignore the wake-up call. I wanted to see my episode literally and metaphorically. I was afforded an opportunity to untangle my "inner laundry" before the washing machine broke down or the contents became so tightly knotted that they were impossible to unravel. I had let go of what I didn't even appreciate that I was holding onto and hiding. I looked and listened anew after my unacknowledged exhaustion made it impossible to ignore what was happening.

Stop, Look, and Listen

"Stop, look, and listen." Isn't this what we have been instructed to do at corners, turns, and crossroads since we were children? The advice is still useful. I stop, look, and listen regularly. My vacation time allowed me to stop—fortunately, before a health crisis made the stop mandatory. During this period, I asked myself the four self-assessment questions in chapter 1 many times. What was I thinking about obligation and duty that kept me working longer hours and more days than were consistent with getting enough rest and relaxation? What was I feeling about loyalty and guilt and security that moved me out of healthy balance? How were my priorities, limits, and boundaries working? Was I being driven forward or held back by fear? Fear of what? Failure, loss of control, insufficiency? I took stock repeatedly and redefined where I was, how I had gotten there, and where I needed to go. I asked how I could correct my course on my own and where I needed help.

Upon returning to work, I restructured my schedule to allow at least some time on a weekly basis to do what I needed to do to "rest at the oars." I stopped carrying as much work home at night. I gave up a formal briefcase and resorted to a canvas bag to serve as a ready reminder of my goal. I started carrying both hiking boots and a yoga mat and clothes in the car so I could take advantage of an opportunity for some downtime at the spur of the moment. Because my training as a physician has contributed to a long-standing dedication to service and overwork, I knew I would need help in following through on my desired changes, so I enlisted the support of my staff and my family.

Review the schedule, rebalance the workload, and ensure that time is available for solitude, contemplation, and quiet time with family. Revisit yearnings, motivations, fears, and insecurities, and ensure priorities and pacing that are sustainable. That is what I did then and what all of us must do regularly to begin or sustain our path to well-being.

If you're dealing with only the external or superficial (symptoms) without identifying associated, underlying aspects (emotions, needs, desires, beliefs), you have a much lower likelihood of succeeding in making changes. Your self-assessment (diagnosis) and treatment plan (healing changes) must be accurate and honest, or you won't be a valuable healer for yourself or for others. Your challenge and your responsibility are to take stock regularly of where you are and to measure your "vital signs": your physical, mental, emotional, and spiritual well-being. When you find imbalances and disconnections between where you are and where you want to be, obstacles that stand in the way of yearnings, you must pay attention and correct your course, preferably before you find yourself in a crisis.

LASTING CHANGE

A patient was diagnosed with a chronic viral liver disease. The illness catalyzed a change in her philosophic viewpoint and stimulated an honest evaluation of the meaning and purpose of her life. Once she recognized the overpowering level of stress in her life, she was able to begin to bring balance to her daily existence. This required that she make life-changing decisions, but given her diagnosis, the pain of staying the same was greater than her fear of changing. She was able to shift her goals from her business life to her inner life, starting with small steps. For example, she began a meditation practice and initially meditated while lying down, then progressed to standing meditation to define what she was willing to stand up for, and then to walking meditation for problem solving. As she integrated small steps into her daily life, they led to sustainable changes. Eventually she began taking a yoga class. As her insights deepened and her physical status strengthened, the results from these shifts served as ongoing motivators.

Not only were her human values affected, her lab values reflected her holistic therapy. The complementary medicine practices in partnership with her conventional care resulted in a reduction of her viral load from thirty-two million to undetectable over a brief period. She now calls her illness a life-changing gift.

Changing requires you to plumb your depths honestly. Your health-creating decisions must go beyond undergoing treatment for a chronic illness, changing your job, finding a new life partner, or joining a support group. Each of these acts may be part of a healthful, constructive shift, but lasting change requires deep questioning, self-discovery, and ongoing discipline, commitment, and course correction, otherwise your changes may be hollow, short-lived gestures designed to gain approval, acceptance, advancement, or safe harbor. They won't serve your core needs unless they are based on truth telling and personal authenticity. Cover-ups don't lead to meaningful, sustainable progress on your healing path. Your willingness to change must be deeply rooted and persevering, because it will be challenged many times along the way. If you set the footings properly, with a personal philosophy that is strong and flexible and tools to help guide you (more on this in chapter 3), you'll be better prepared as each challenge or obstacle appears on your path.

EXERCISES FOR CHAPTER 2: BREAKDOWN OR BREAKTHROUGH?

Exercise 1: Questions for Self-Inquiry

The work of self-inquiry, self-assessment, and self-discovery doesn't have to be bitter medicine that's hard to swallow. It is deep medicine, which leads to healing at a fundamental level. To begin to build a foundation for health and change and to identify aspects of your life that may be calling for a shift, ask yourself the following questions:

- Why am I here?

- What are some of the milestone events that have led me to where I am today?

- What is the meaning of my life?

- What is the purpose of my life?

- Am I living in ways that are consistent with the meaning and purpose of my life?

- What is my calling?

- What are the values that govern my life?

- What is my life's dream?

- What are my gifts and my talents? How can I bring them forward?

- What do I need?

- What are the resources available to me?

- What obstacles do I currently face?

- What can I do to begin to effect change and move toward my goals in the next...

    - Twenty-four hours?

    - One week?

    - One month?

    - Six months?

    - One year?

    - Five years?

Answering questions like these is challenging. It requires honesty and causes discomfort. We all want to look good, and we all want to avoid discomfort or get past it quickly. The hard questions seem poorly defined and unanswerable. We would welcome some multiple-choice options.

As you practice self-inquiry and become more comfortable with the process, it will get easier. You'll realize that the answers are less important than asking good questions. A good question is more relevant to learning and growth than a seemingly right answer. So continue to inquire in the spirit of the good question. The specific questions and answers will change, but the work of authentic inquiry will offer ongoing rewards.

Exercise 2: Identifying Your Stressors

In which of the following domains of life are you feeling stressed, and what are your identifiable stressors in each realm?

- Health

- Relationships

- Work

- Sense of abundance, prosperity, or resources

Having identified specific stressors, you're in a better position to devise a plan for both external and internal stress management.

Exercise 3: Reviewing Your Projects for Change

At any given time, we are involved in multiple self-improvement projects in the change process. Select several of your personal rebalancing projects and take inventory of them. Can you categorize your projects as to which classic stage of change each is in at the present time? Which of the four core competencies would best serve your progress in each at this time?

Start by naming your highest priority project as clearly and with as few words as possible. Consider why you chose it: because it was easiest, the most likely to succeed, the most critical to your health, or something else? Whatever the reason, use this issue to begin a pilot project with yourself. Be sure you are ready, motivated, and confident, then embark on the journey toward making this change. Keep a journal to record your progress, challenges, and results—including both successes and setbacks.

Be creative. Try to link things you like to do with things you need to do. For example, link dancing and exercise, combine being with your family with being out in nature, or use your desire to make your home or garden a sacred space to help you clear out clutter or an unkempt weed patch. Enhancing your environment, in all of its manifestations, can be a great stimulus for growth in energy, health, and contentment.

What does your talk tell you about your likelihood of changing? Is it change talk or resistance talk?

Exercise 4: Where Is Your Resistance?

Most often the biggest hurdle to change is moving from awareness of an issue or problem to taking real action in a committed way. In other words, the blockage occurs between becoming aware of the desired change and commitment to taking action to change.

Can you identify and target your resistance or blockage in the cascade of stages of change for health-creating activities? Can you identify the point in the stages of change where you are resisting, and the source of your resistance, such as certain fears or beliefs that prevent you from starting or continuing health-creating activities? For example, you might believe you aren't strong or healthy enough to begin the process of change, or that you don't have the time to implement needed changes.

Are you aware of what you want to change? Are you acting on your desired changes? Are you integrating the changes you are making into your daily life?

CHAPTER 3

Tools for Change

By a single thought that comes into mind, in one moment,
a hundred worlds are overturned.

—Rumi

We can rise above our limitations,
only once we recognize them.

—B. K. S. Iyengar

As you arrive at an understanding of the change process and its relationship to your health and well-being, you move from establishing a knowledge base to the acquisition of skills. Through your behavior, you begin to apply what you have learned as theory, fact, or philosophy. Your progress moves from thought and feeling to word and act, then, ultimately, to habit and character development. Consciousness changes, actions change, and character changes. You will need tools to effect these changes. The tools for change explored in this chapter are naming, symbols and images, stories and myths, dreams, and teachers.

As you progress along the stages of change, how you describe or name a condition, desired outcome, or goal has tremendous power and carries great meaning. Identifying, observing, describing, naming, and tracking are early and ongoing necessities if you intend to change something. Using the medical model as an example, medically based inquiry is usually focused on the chief complaint and on the history related to recent and past episodes of sickness. It may be useful to expand the medical model of inquiry to include people's full story, not just their symptoms and history. Only then can a medical diagnosis capture the full context and scope of the condition presenting to the physician as a medical problem. When a doctor makes a diagnosis, a naming is taking place. The accuracy of that naming is of utmost importance, as it determines the action steps, or treatment plan, that will follow.

YOUR PERSONAL BALANCING ACT

What can you learn from the medical model about your own self-assessment? How can you capture your wholeness as you name your desired changes, and in so doing influence the effectiveness of the actions you take and tools you use for your own healing? Your healing must be a personal balancing act. In the process, you will right your inner and outer gyroscopes again and again in response to both internal and external circumstances, which are constantly changing in ways both predictable and, more often, unpredictable. You must heed and respond to your internal world, as manifested in awareness, consciousness, thoughts, feelings, emotions, dreams, and more, and external circumstances related to work, your environment, relationships, economic factors, and so on.

The same level of precision needed for a useful diagnosis is necessary when you name your values and goals in regard to enhancement of health, self-development, rebalancing, and change. This naming, be it literal or metaphoric, must consider the full topography of your landscape—physical, emotional, mental, and spiritual. For example, the diagnosis of heart disease for chest pain due to narrowed arteries supplying blood to the heart doesn't indicate in what other ways a person's heart may be broken, closed, weak, or less than whole. Because it is necessary to address all things that impact our well-being, our inner needs and desires are as important to the naming of our ailments as the anatomy and physiology that usually define our maladies. It is mandatory that you discover and harness the healing power you carry as part of your quest for well-being. Health issues, which often have hidden inner causes, cannot be fully resolved with solutions that are strictly external. If you don't awaken and engage your inner healing potential, you are overlooking a vast source of healing power.

WHAT'S IN A NAME?

Whereas we understand that the menu is not the meal and the map is not the territory, mere mention of many words catalyzes a response as full-blown as the actual thing. What happens at the mention of rotten eggs, for example, or Mom's apple pie? Halloween? These words trigger thoughts, emotions, and memories that have physiologic consequences for our minds and bodies. Most of us would rather dive into an activity described as a piece of cake than one referred to as a tough nut to crack. We would rather hike the trail called Morning Glory than one designated Widow Maker, regardless of the actual nature of the terrain.

In relationship to health and well-being, Westerners have typically conceived of health care in two ways: as a battlefield and as a marketplace. Both of these metaphors have powerful implications for medical diagnosis and treatment, and for how we name our personal conditions and choose tools for their management.

The Battlefield

In the battlefield metaphor, disease is the enemy; doctors, nurses, and other health care professionals are soldiers; and our bodies are the battleground. We employ an arsenal of medications and technology to wage war against cancer, fight heart disease, and wipe out resistant infections, advancing battle lines and frontiers in the process. These harsh images are often difficult to accept when dealing with infirmity, death, or the birthing of new life.

Early in my surgical career, I operated on a lovely woman with a large malignant tumor located next to and behind one of her eyes. The surgery was very extensive, requiring the removal of her eye and all of the tissues around it in her eye socket. It was an aggressive operation to stop an aggressive malignancy. Fortunately, the tumor was completely removed surgically.

Because of the risk of local recurrence, the group of specialists who reviewed her case recommended radiation therapy but not chemotherapy as part of her postsurgical medical management. At an early postoperative visit with my patient, I described the successful results of the surgery and the expert panel's recommendations. I discussed the battle plan with the intention of conveying the positive aspects of the treatment plan and prognosis in this very serious situation.

Two days later, the patient's sister called me saying the patient had been devastated by our visit. Her sister wanted to know what had happened. I had conveyed the plan of attack and expressed that we were in a good place in very tough circumstances. My patient, however, had interpreted the fact that there was no need to do chemotherapy as there being no possibility of containing the tumor, rather than there was no added benefit to adding chemotherapy in light of the complete surgical removal of the tumor and the added effect of the planned radiation therapy. Unintentionally, I had taken away her hope by describing which treatment weapons and battle tactics we thought most likely to win the war against her cancer. My sensitivity to the battlefield metaphor was forever changed, and since that time, I've worked to ensure that hope is always carefully woven into the description of any prognosis and treatment plan.

Although the image of the good fight has an important place in our healing vocabulary, the best generals often win by negotiation. The best healers are not necessarily those running about attempting to cure disease, but the little-seen practitioners who focus on preventing illness. In *The Art of War* (1991), legendary Chinese warrior and philosopher Sun Tzu draws parallels between the healing arts and the martial arts. In both, naming the problem is the key to solutions. He demonstrates that disharmony and change are integral to both realms. Being a master of balance, he teaches that ideal strategies accomplish the most by doing less early, rather than by doing more later—a concept familiar to us in the adage "An ounce of prevention is worth a pound of cure." He advises being discerning and prudent yet willing to take calculated risks, but not needless ones, and that to win without fighting is best. He advocates adapting to situations the way water flows over changing contours and a river meanders to overcome obstacles.

You can learn a great deal about your path toward well-being from this ancient wisdom and the unexpected similarities between the healing arts and the martial arts. Yielding and retreat, not just pushing relentlessly forward, may be necessary as part of a larger plan and deeper purpose. The art of war is a tool for understanding the roots of conflict and its resolution. Similarly, deep medicine is an approach to understanding health and healing.

The Marketplace

In the second metaphor, the marketplace, health is a commodity. What this means is that health becomes an article of trade or commerce. Patients become consumers and clients, and their lives and health are managed on an economic basis. Hospitals and clinics become providers, while insurance companies and health maintenance organizations become payers. In this picture, lines of revenue, cost centers, quarterly profits, and methods of accounting come to dominate.

We must acknowledge the cost of our health care practices, but we can't allow these fiscal implications to overshadow our needs as humans. The fiscal and material constraints on our health and healing practices are real and must be incorporated into affordable practices, but finances alone cannot be permitted to drive a realm so fraught with the complexities of being human. We must still compassionately care for the very young, very old, and very sick.

Ecology—A New Metaphor for Health

Though useful, both the battlefield and the marketplace metaphors for health and healing are limiting. For a complete vision of health, we need a new metaphor that incorporates a fresh vocabulary and new reference points for health. As George Annas, professor of health law, bioethics, and human rights, aptly put it, "If Congress is ever to make meaningful progress in reforming our fast-changing system for financing and delivering medical care, a new way must be found to think about health itself. This will require at least a new metaphoric framework that permits us to re-envision and thus to reconstruct the American medical care system. I suggest that the leading candidate for a new metaphor is ecology" (1995, p. 746).

When an ecologic metaphor for medicine is employed, disease is seen as an imbalance; the work of the physician, nurse, and health practitioner is stewardship; the hospital is part of the ecosystem; and healing becomes part of the process of change, or adaptation. With the wisdom of nature as a guide, the ecology metaphor offers a workable and sustainable approach to health that acknowledges key principles such as evolution (that we are in a continuous, dynamic state of change), interdependence (that our existence is part of a larger web of life), limits (that our resources are bounded, not infinite), diversity (that every part of the whole is unique and makes an essential contribution), and cycles (that we are a part of nature's patterns and rhythms). (This model is adapted from the Center for Ecoliteracy 2008.)

I like this metaphor for health and for change because it speaks to fundamental processes that underlie all aspects of our existence. Ecology is the study of the relationships among living organisms and their environments, and ecological systems are driven by evolution—the process of change over time. In the 4.6 billion years since the Earth formed, climates have changed, landmasses have moved, and species have come and gone. Change is our reality.

Ecology as a metaphor for health and medicine has deep roots, going back at least to the 1700s, when physician and geologist James Hutton proposed the specialty of planetary medicine. Hutton thought species-specific medicine—medical practices dealing only with the human species—was too small in scope, and that if we don't take into consideration all else that coexists with us on the planet, we can't properly diagnose or treat any malady. As you shall read in chapter 6, Hutton's perspective is even more relevant today than when proposed centuries ago.

WE'RE ALL IN IT TOGETHER

The ecology metaphor reminds us we're all in it together and offers us a chance to come to terms with the transitory nature of health. The whole and its parts must be seen in a both-and context, not as an either-or duality. Our personal little picture and the larger big picture need to be viewed simultaneously—ecologically. Push here, something bulges over there. Pour toxic waste into the sewer, and it shows up in the bay to be consumed in a future seafood buffet. Overgraze a field, and the soil will erode; the stock will subsequently go hungry, as will the human population waiting for them to go to market. (Chapter 7 discusses becoming whole, with this metaphor in mind.)

Because everything is connected, subtle changes may lead to large disruptions. A tiny plaque in a coronary artery can cause a massive heart attack. A small embolus lodged in a blood vessel in the brain can result in a stroke, or "brain attack." A minimal change in water quality or quantity can upset plant and animal productivity and health. Relatedness isn't confined to a specific location. Our common ancestry and humanity link us over great distances. In a sense, our compassion for the starving in Africa or the sick in India has roots in our shared origins and planetary linkages.

Every part of the whole matters. Our bodies require a diverse population of cells, tissues, and organs. All are essential to our healthy functioning. Brain, heart, muscle, bone, and blood—all must work in concert toward the greater good. This is holistic medicine; this is deep medicine. Recognizing the value of variation in the natural world can help us value the diversity of human experience, background, culture, race, age, opinions, and solutions. When we are open to multiple possibilities, we find more options on our own path to health.

Just as exhalation follows inhalation, digestion follows ingestion, night follows day, and death follows life, our existence is a part of nature's cyclical patterns. Every moment, we experience the pumping of the heart, the flow of the blood, and the rhythm of our breathing. On an ecological level, the planetary pulse brings us the cycles of night and day, the movement of the moon around the Earth, and the seasonal variations of winter, spring, summer, and fall, with their attendant preparation, budding, blooming, and harvest. The cycles of birth, growth, aging, death, and decay are natural phenomena to be understood and accepted. The same patterns of endings, new beginnings, and transitions fill our personal and professional lives.

The ecology metaphor offers the breadth and depth needed to truly understand health and create new healing practices. It doesn't imply we'll be free of difficult decisions, challenges to our understanding, or the need to compromise, nor does it mean that everyone will be satisfied or happy all the time. It does, however, provide useful perspective for meeting the challenges of creating personal health and contributing to the well-being of the world around us.

SYMBOLS AND IMAGES FOR HEALING

Gandhi taught that most of what we do will seem insignificant, but it is essential that we do it, and that we be the change we want to see in the world.

Change requires movement—action that carries you toward something you want or away from something you don't want. Although change may occur suddenly, it generally takes a long time. Each of us has our own personal cadence of discovery and activity. We march to our own rhythm. For some, change may occur in one giant step. But little steps, often separated by long plateaus, are more likely. Doing a little bit every day is a good approach. Many of the steps might not seem particularly significant when they occur, but upon reflection, they may be seen as pivotal moves. A true shift will begin with the dawning of awareness and sincere, honest self-inquiry.

Accurate naming and appropriate metaphors serve to define us and our needs so we can act accordingly. The following tools can serve you well on the path to health. They foster both change and movement, and allow you to move forward at your own pace with conscious self-discovery. They are sources of health and healing. They allow you to create your own to-do list.

The Labyrinth

When working with people seeking to change their health status, I find the labyrinth a helpful tool for catalyzing change. The labyrinth is a representation of step-by-step advancement along a path connecting outside to inside. Some forms have dead ends and therefore are mazes, but in most labyrinths you won't get lost, because there is a well-defined, although convoluted, path into the center and back out again. The path often turns back on itself, and you frequently can't see exactly where you're going. Symbolically, it demonstrates a route to an inner destination and then back out to where you began.

The labyrinth is a powerful symbol of the union of your inner and outer work on the path to health and healing. Your symptoms, thoughts, feelings, and actions—from recurring patterns of behavior to acute and chronic signs and symptoms of illness—can be engaged using this practical working model capable of accommodating your physical, psychological, emotional, behavioral, spiritual, and mythological dimensions.

The labyrinth can symbolize a path to your psychological or mythological source or center. It can be a metaphor for seeking your inner or core issues that relate to outer behavior or symptoms. You start on the outside, amidst your habits, behaviors, symptoms, and stories, and work your way to your interior, where you encounter underlying causes and core issues. Within your deepest self, you can discover wisdom, beliefs, fears, and character traits that underlie your external behavior, personality, or symptoms. Are you holding yourself back out of fear of failing, succeeding, or being seen? Is your pain related to unexpressed anger or resentment? Is there someone you need to forgive? Is it yourself?

Your journey in the labyrinth is not complete once you reach the center of the inner circle. You must then return to the outside. You take your wisdom, your discoveries, your changes, and your treasure from the walk inward and return to the place on the outside of the circle where you began. Here your inner rewards can be applied in the external world. Did your honest assessment in the imposed quiet of the labyrinth reveal a secret or a solution? Have issues around scarcity and survival manifested in you in such a way as to limit your capacity for generosity and sharing? Do you have a desire for control that leads to frequent disagreements with colleagues? Do you fear an early death, associated with the diagnosis of cancer in a family member at a young age, catalyzing a fear of every ache and pain, resulting in excessive visits to the doctor, and preventing you from living your life fully?

As with all tools and symbols, you must be cautious not to romanticize the labyrinth as solely a path to treasure and self-discovery. The labyrinth can also symbolize the path taken again and again—the rut. As you contemplate change, ask yourself what the payoff is that keeps you attached to your present behavior patterns or perspective. Assessing this honestly will help clarify the next obstacle to overcome along your chosen path.

Oracle-Based Wisdom

Another way people seek guidance is with various forms of oracle-based wisdom, such as astrology, Tarot cards, animal medicine cards, angel cards, the I Ching hexagrams, tea leaves, palmistry, and other age-old practices for seeking answers to life's questions. Perhaps the most common form of this activity in everyday use is the horoscope, often found in magazines and in the daily newspaper. Although these practices are often labeled "new age," they are anything but new. Many have been used for thousands of years by many people from many cultures.

When you use these techniques, you need to trust the wisdom that leads you to hear what you hear or to choose the card that you select—or that selects you. Then you must be curious and flexible in the way that you interpret how it may apply to your individual circumstances. Some of the messages you find could be applied, in a generic way, to almost anyone, so many people dismiss the information that comes from these sources. Nonetheless, there is always some applicable wisdom to be found, even if it feels totally contrary to your present situation.

STORIES AND MYTHS

Much wisdom is embodied in the oral and written traditions of great cultures and peoples. We are continuously surrounded by stories: life stories, news stories, bedtime stories, books, movies, stories told by family and friends about the dramas of daily life. Stories can be healing and transforming and serve as valuable tools for describing and inspiring movement as they create openings for change. They can also immobilize us by diverting us from the untidy and sometimes painful work of self-investigation. In the form of myth, they provide access to a domain of experiences much larger than our individual lives and carry us deep below the surface reality of our existence.

Always consider what you can learn from the stories you hear and tell. There is always something to learn. And remember, in six months you may feel very differently about a story you hear today. As you listen, consider the perspective of the teller and also appreciate that your viewpoint or interpretation may be different.

Personal Stories

We can get stuck in personal stories, repeating them time and again to gain sympathy and acceptance. This behavior is an impediment to growth and healing. In a related vein, it is crucial to avoid the pitfall of blaming, faultfinding, or being a victim in your stories. Always carefully observe what stories evoke—what memories, sensations, emotions, bodily responses, and even dreams come up in response to hearing your own or another's story. Listen, but listen carefully. Guard against being distracted or put off, and against comparing your story to someone else's. As your personal story, it is incomparable! The rule of the road here is that comparison is rarely valid; it gains you nothing real.

Your stories are important not only to you, but to those who hear them. This is particularly true when the story reveals aspects of your inner world and is not just another description, narrative, or travelogue about your outer world. You never know what someone else's story will catalyze in you, or when the telling of your own story will open a door for someone else. When someone tells you a story, listen not just to the words, but also for the message beneath the words. Listening only to the surface narrative is like trying to tell a book by its cover, which we know we cannot do. Don't fables always have a moral? Would you buy a house only because of its curb appeal, without going inside? Would you buy a car without driving it? Whether by reading between the lines or listening to the spaces in the silence between words, you must be alert and present to fully learn what a story holds for you. Those stories that truly resonate probably hold a particularly valuable message that may not be apparent at first. We'll explore further the value of stories as sources of your healing power in chapter 5.

Shared Stories

You don't exist in a vacuum. As you travel your personal journey, you must acknowledge fellow travelers—the groups and communities in which you exist and which powerfully influence you. Everyone has ancestors and lineage. You are a part of a nuclear family, the family of humanity, and the community of all living beings. You are "star stuff" and part of the continuum from subatomic particles to atoms, molecules, cells, organs, and organisms. You are a citizen of a town, state, and country. You are part of a society, a culture, and possibly a religion. You are formed and defined in part by your genetic heritage and your socioeconomic status.

Beyond your individual work, your personal quest for balance and wholeness must acknowledge and address your relationships within the many groups with which you are intimately involved and by which you are knowingly and unknowingly influenced. Do you live your parents' stories and dreams, or your own? Have you adapted your life to society's dictates, or have you followed your own passions? Your personal story and your changes on an individual level are only part of the fabric of the collectives to which you belong, but they are an extremely important part. Everyone is part of the critical mass necessary to effect large-scale change.

DREAMS AND DREAMING

Your inner and outer work are inseparable. Dreams are a source of great inner guidance and wisdom, and a powerful tool in the process of change and healing. The actual definition of dream is quite broad. To dream is to consider, conceive, or imagine something. In certain stages of sleep, dreams manifest as images, emotions, and ideas. Daydreams may take the form of reverie or trance. A dream may be a deeply desired aspiration or something extremely beautiful or pleasant. A dreamer is one inclined to interpret experience with imagination and without strict regard to practical concerns.

Because external activity is suspended as you sleep, dreams give your subconscious mind an opportunity to connect with your inner world. In your dreams, you may be visited by allies in human, animal, or other forms. The knowledge they impart during your dreaming life can help illuminate your waking life. Being attentive to these messages, perhaps even recording them, can unlock a powerful source of insight. You might even try to harness it. Sometime when you're dealing with a thorny dilemma, try posing a question about it before you go to sleep. Ask for some input to come your way during your sleep, then pay attention to any information you receive through your dreams.

During his midlife crisis, psychiatrist Carl Jung discovered that he didn't know by which myth he was living (his life dream, if you will), so he made it an urgent life task to find out. When poet Donald Hall met with sculptor Henry Moore, he dared to ask Moore if he believed there was a secret to life. Moore responded that the secret to life is to have a task that you devote your entire life to—something so big that you bring everything to it. What was most important, though, was that it had to be something that you could not possibly do (Cousineau 1998). Your dreams must be big enough to hold the expanse of your inner self. If your dreams are too small, they will create a container too limited for your full flowering.

Dreams are a tool for well-being because they fortify you for the dynamic balancing act required for the lifelong establishing and maintaining of your health. You need to identify your dreams and longings, and you need to pursue them. Your dreams give you the energy for manifesting in the world. Your conscious awareness and inner life are the sources for your outer deeds and actions. If you aren't in touch with your dreams and longings, it's very difficult to sustain healthy progress on the path of well-being. Being in alignment with your deepest dreams and passions gives you an energy and endurance for the outer journey that you cannot derive from willfulness, stubbornness, determination, or material rewards. When you're sustained from within, you will tire less easily and persist more happily in your quest. When you are healthy, your inner and outer purposes are aligned.

I had a dream to create a healing center within contemporary, establishment medicine. I dreamed of a place that served aspects of healing that weren't necessarily visible and spoke to the needs of patients and practitioners around compassion, caring, comfort, and coping. While contemporary medicine has been very efficient in dealing with the science, mechanics, and technology of disease and treatment, it has not been as effective at acknowledging and managing the fears, worry, dependency, and isolation of patients associated with their illness. Nor has it readily acknowledged or learned from alternative sources that can contribute to healing. Therefore, I dreamed of a center that supported practitioners who saw and served both the inner and outer aspects of illness and healing in each person—a center that fostered well-being and recovery with its very design, decor, and atmosphere.

This dream of a real healing community was a possibility first born in my imagination. The manifestation of my dream occurred through commitment, discipline, hard work, and the support of many others. Just as hope and courage connect our past shortcomings, failures, and learnings with the possibilities of the future, our dreamtime creativity connects our inner consciousness, dreams, and thoughts with action in the external world.

It is from your dreams that the fire to fight the good fight of your life comes. Your dreams must be healing stories, not recurring nightmares or negative tales, so that they can provide nourishment for your inner healer, just as a meal does for the physical body. Never stop dreaming, no matter how many times in your life you see your dreams shattered or frustrated.

What is the dream plan for your life?

TEACHERS

A Chinese proverb states that teachers can open the door, but you must enter by yourself. No one can answer your questions for you. No teacher, workshop, or book, no matter how good, can eliminate the time, work, and sweat of your own self-inquiry. Only through the hard work of gaining self-knowledge by means of exploration, experimentation, trials, and tribulations—the mindful experiencing and processing of what comes your way—will you gain the insights to guide your actions and define your values on the path toward your life dream. This does not mean teachers are unimportant. They are critical for anyone's progress. However, no single teacher will provide all of the wisdom and training that you need over time. Many will touch you for varying periods, but in the end it's up to you.

When you're ready, teachers will appear, and they probably won't be garbed in robes or speak in homilies. Rather, you will find them in the checkout line, on the freeway, or in the office. Their lessons may be subtle or in-your-face. Treating everyone, even a rival, as your teacher can lead to profound learning and health-creating changes.

Don't overlook the possibility of being your own teacher. Waiting passively for a sudden shift stimulated by an external teacher or guide makes little sense if you're responding to rumblings within that beckon you to heal. You can choose to embark on a path to shift your perception in a health-generating direction on your own. Take yourself to your own personal school of self-knowledge and complete your homework. Your first study session will require little more than a quiet place and a brief period of uninterrupted time to begin to pursue an intimacy with yourself. Allow this first date to evolve into a daily appointment with yourself as you explore your heartfelt desires and needs. In these interludes, you will be both patient and healer.

USE THE TOOLS!

You likely have noticed that the tools of change described above are somewhat universal, as opposed to laying out specific plans or modalities to address specific conditions. This universality is intentional and makes them applicable to your specific needs and desires. You have the latitude and the responsibility to apply them in the ways that best suit you. This may involve customized nutrition plans, exercise programs, or contemplative practices, depending on what attracts you as your next health-creating step.

What you must appreciate about tools (and there are many others beyond those noted here) is that in order for them to contribute to change and healing, they must be used! Many of us are very good at collecting tools, plans, and programs from many sources but are less capable or motivated when it comes to using those tools. Many tools for change are time-tested, of known effectiveness, and evidence based. However, if you don't use them or practice what you've learned, your skills won't improve and you won't realize your potential. Understand that this has reverberations beyond you and your life. Through your personal work of change and healing, your personal growth influences your intimate contacts and your communities. As you change, your world changes. Your personal wellness contributes to the greater good and to planetary healing.

Several categories of tools for change have been described in this chapter: metaphors, symbols and images, stories, dreams, and teachers. In each category there are many possibilities. How then do you choose the best tools for your personal self-improvement project? This requires honest self-assessment to ascertain both what is alluring and what is available. Explore and experiment to match the tool to your needs. What arouses your curiosity or your passion? What feels right? What brings you joy? What works, and what doesn't?

EXERCISES FOR CHAPTER 3: CHOOSING AND USING THE BEST TOOLS FOR YOU

Exercise 1: Explore Metaphor

Metaphor involves comparison and is the application of a descriptor to an object or a concept that it doesn't literally describe. Explore the ecologic metaphor for health by considering a health-related condition you're presently experiencing or a health-related change you're considering or actually making. How do the following aspects relate to your condition or desired change?

- **Evolution:** When, where, and how did your situation or desired change originate and how has it progressed?

- **Interdependence:** How is it related to aspects of your life such as work, relationship, and sense of security?

- **Limits:** How has it affected your activities of daily life, what you can and can't do for yourself, and how independent or dependent you are?

- **Diversity:** What unique contribution is it making to your progress on your life's path? And how does it relate to the many threads contributing to the fabric of your life?

- **Cycles:** How does it relate to where you are in various aspects of your growth and development? What bearing does it have on how you are being challenged, surprised, or inspired at this time? What season does it seem to be in your life?

Exercise 2: Explore Your Stories About Your Health

Recall a story that you tell yourself and others about your health. Is it a healing story or a horror story? If it isn't a healing story, how can you change it to make it into one? Review the stories below as related by Olympic runner Bill Mills in his book *Wokini*. They are the "Eight Lies of Iktomi," the trickster or liar figure from the Lakota tradition. Each of these stories can set up obstacles in a person's life and jeopardize happiness and well-being (1999, p. 45):

1. If only I were rich, then I would be happy.

2. If only I were famous, then I would be happy.

3. If only I could find the right person to marry, then I would be happy.

4. If only I had more friends, then I would be happy.

5. If only I were more attractive, then I would be happy.

6. If only I weren't physically handicapped in any way, then I would be happy.

7. If only someone close to me hadn't died, then I would be happy.

8. If only the world were a better place, then I would be happy.

None of these stories is true in relationship to our happiness and salvation. We obsessively strive for as many of the eight illusions as we can; however, once these goals are attained, we are often stunned to find ourselves still wishing for satisfaction, meaning, or happiness. Only by ceasing to strive can we be liberated from our fear, false attachments, and desires.

Take some time to reflect on which of the eight lies have driven your personal and professional expression in different areas of your life, and how this has ultimately impacted you.

Exercise 3: Explore a Labyrinth

Seek out a full-size walking labyrinth near your home or obtain a finger labyrinth. Walk or trace your path into and out of the labyrinth, noting the three stages of the process described (1995) by the Reverend Lauren Artress of Grace Cathedral in San Francisco and founder of Veriditas: The Worldwide Labyrinth Project.

1. **Releasing:** Entering the labyrinth and shedding thoughts and distractions, quiet your mind and open your heart.

2. **Receiving:** Reach the center and receive what is there for you to receive.

3. **Returning:** Leave the center, following the same path by which you entered, to join with the healing forces at work in the world.

Having completed the three steps described by Reverend Artress, *reflect* on what you experienced and learned and how you might integrate your discoveries into your daily life.

Exercise 4: Remember a Mentor

Recall an important teacher, coach, or mentor in each decade of your life and the lessons you learned from each. Have you still found inspiration or guidance in their teachings over time? Is there a pattern to the lessons? What teachings apply to the present time and circumstances for you? Are you still making progress with what you have learned, or are you stuck?

Exercise 5: Explore Your Dreams

Do you have a dream, passion, or calling that you are following? What are you doing to bring it to fruition? What keeps you from acting on your dream? What resources do you need to pursue your inner calling or outer purpose, and what resources do you already have? Think of a small daily action that would forward the realization of your current dream, for example, giving gratitude, setting intentions, making a plan, seeking information, signing up for a class, or collecting images and making a collage that reflects your dream. Then commit to taking that action.

Exercise 6: Explore Your Thoughts

Consider the following words from Buddha: "The thought manifests as the word; the word manifests as the deed; the deed develops into habit; and habit hardens into character. So watch the thought and its ways with care, and let it spring from love born out of concern for all beings."

Take time to consider the meaning of this statement and how you can apply it to your thoughts, words, deeds, habits, and character.

CHAPTER 4

Pillars and Practices
of Self-Care

If you want to change the world, first change yourself.
And when you are changed, truly changed, everything
around you will be changed.

—Sign posted on the wall at the Sri Aurobindo ashram

You cannot solve a problem with the same level of
thinking that created it.

—Albert Einstein

As we gain insight and perspective, we are challenged to act. Practical, sustainable actions move us along the healing path. In this chapter, you will plot a course of personal action. You will create a customized plan for your health and healing using principles and practices that can initiate and sustain your desired health-creating changes.

The first three chapters established a conceptual foundation on which to base health-creating choices and changes. This foundation is compatible with objectivity and science. It also sets a context that incorporates beliefs, values, and intuition. It isn't a simple, unchanging recipe for better health; it's a database that provides resources to be used as needed. As you move forward on your healing path, here are some basic guidelines to keep in mind:

- Be curious and willing to change.

- Consider your connection to all around you and to the greater good. That is, consider the impact of what you do, beyond yourself and on those close to you.

- Be open to bridging what might appear to be contradictions.

- Tell your authentic life story to yourself and others.

- Remember that your inner world needs as much attention as your outer world.

- Be generous with yourself. Small steps are okay—and sometimes mandatory.

- Your progress deserves acknowledgment and celebration. Emphasize and acknowledge what you *did* do, not just what you didn't do!

- Always remember that you are in this for the long haul and not just the short run.

- Above all else, don't forget that everything you think, feel, say, or do either contributes to creating your health or negates it.

In this chapter, we will explore the four pillars of self-care: nutrition, physical activity and relaxation, relationship and community, and contemplation and solitude. Self-care provides the support structure for your health and well-being. Although self-care isn't the only determinant of your health, your self-care choices and actions present a powerful opportunity to influence recovery from illness, prevention of disease, maximum performance, optimal aging, and all other aspects of your health. Learning to apply self-care practices successfully is part of practicing deep medicine. We will also engage four practices for realizing and harnessing your healing power: slowing down, getting quiet, paying attention, and going inward.

Self-care is not simply about what you do; it's also about how you do it. It is about your inner being as well as your outer doing— about your thoughts, emotions, and spirituality as well as your physical actions. Therefore, as you consider the four pillars and the four practices, you will be merging your outer, external circumstances and your inner world and deeper self.

THE HEART OF DEEP MEDICINE

We are moving into the heart of the work of deep medicine: the place where your aspirations meet your need for action. Both your attention and your intention are required to keep you fully present, as your character will be challenged by the need for honesty, patience, flexibility, commitment, determination, and persistence. Sometimes your progress will slow or you may even backslide, and joy and optimism will be displaced by discouragement. Your circumstances, thoughts, and moods will change repeatedly. You must have a substantive inner purpose to support your outer work on yourself and in the world.

Whatever has brought you to this particular starting line—be it a desire to lose weight or prolong your productive lifetime, a bad habit, unfulfilling relationships, an unsatisfying job, loss of direction, a search for meaning and purpose, a distressing illness, or simple curiosity—it is less important than the realization that you must *want* to make a shift. You must deeply and fully want to change. Ultimately, your motivation must come from within, and it must be translated into witnessable action.

In order to sustain growth and change, you must harness them to a meaningful, truthful vision of who you are. This perspective can continually rekindle your inner fire as you encounter challenges. Flexibility, resourcefulness, creativity, commitment, and repeated, determined acts of will are all necessary on your path to health and healing. As you move into making lifestyle changes that the four pillars require, you will bring forward your unique gifts. This will be deeply healing medicine for you and for those around you. Authenticity and truth are always compelling to those who witness them. Let these qualities serve as motivation for you to be unafraid of revealing and expressing who you really are.

As you have probably noticed from reading the previous chapters and doing the exercises, obstacles present themselves, and detours are necessary. They may appear as the family member you enable, the coworker cautioning you, the reluctance to get out of bed for early morning exercise or meditation, the irresistible dessert menu, or the agonizingly slow response to your therapy. You may procrastinate, lose energy, and appear to slip backward. You may stall out, want to quit, need a break, change teachers, seek second and third opinions, and feel fearful.

Yet you will also find inspiration in unlikely places, marveling at the wisdom imparted by seeming strangers, the coincidences that occur, and how what is needed has a way of showing up right on time. Be sensitive to the stage of change that you are in, and stay alert both to your change talk or thoughts and to your resistance talk or thoughts.

SELF-CARE IS PRIMARY CARE

Regardless of your desired destination and your chosen route to it, you must start by taking care of yourself. Although we rarely put our own needs first, this is a mandatory behavior that you must practice repeatedly if you are to be effective in the world and fulfilled in yourself. You can't support your family or your vocation unless you are as healthy as you can be—physically, mentally, emotionally, and spiritually. It is unsustainable to give to others—through obligation, duty, guilt, sacrifice, or other motivation—to the point of burnout. That kind of behavior only contributes to exhaustion and illness.

To make sustainable contributions requires that you do what airlines advise if a serious problem occurs: Put on your own oxygen mask first, then help those around you. It isn't selfish to see to your own well-being first; it is an act of generosity to yourself and to those dependent on you. Don't feel guilty or greedy about it. Only from a foundation of health, wholeness, and balance can you be of service to others.

We are all caregivers—to children, parents, partners, colleagues, friends, neighbors, and the underserved. The need is endless, and you cannot wait until everyone else is taken care of before you bring attention to yourself. Share your energy in a sustainable way, not as a sacrifice, obligation, or responsibility. Share as a gift, in the context of a relationship that serves both giver and receiver. Does this mean you won't get tired, that you won't say yes to too many people? Of course not. But occasional imbalances are temporary in the context of a life plan based on sound self-care principles and practices. Saying no to requests that are health negating will become easier as you recognize your limits and acknowledge your own health needs.

What is essential for your self-care depends on your current state of health and life circumstances. What you do and how you do it will differ according to various cycles and situations. Be creative and proactive as you modify this book's suggestions to suit your own needs. To sustain your self-care, you will probably need expert care as well. Initially, frequent follow-ups with your doctors, healers, coaches, mentors, and guides will serve to sustain your practice and progress toward your goals. Results achieved become ongoing motivators, allowing follow-up intervals to become longer. As your practices become better established, you will wean yourself from your support team and sustain yourself better. However, some type of relational support is essential; never consider it a sign of weakness to check in with your support network as new circumstances arise or for a boost of energy during the long haul.

THE FOUR PILLARS OF SELF-CARE

The endless bookshelves of self-help literature can be condensed into four universal categories of recommendations found in healing systems from multiple cultures. Together, these four pillars create a solid framework of self-care:

1. Nutrition

2. Physical activity and relaxation

3. Relationship and community

4. Contemplation and solitude

These four pillars are literally wisdom practices. They have a deep, well-tested basis in the classic therapies and empirical observations of traditional and indigenous cultures worldwide. They occur in various forms in different cultures as part of inclusive systems (for example, traditional Chinese medicine and ayurveda) that also incorporate guidelines regarding morals, ethics, and acceptable behaviors toward ancestors and elders. In the West, with our quick-fix orientation, we often see yoga only as exercise postures (asanas) and neglect the well-defined recommendations and teachings that underlie the practice. We whittle down the wisdom of generations of Chinese medicine practitioners to only acupuncture or acupressure without consideration of the greater context in which the practice dwells.

These origins of the four pillars are exemplified by millennia-old writings in the *Yellow Emperor's Classic of Internal Medicine*, which sound as relevant today as up-to-date contemporary research findings do:

> *In the past, people practiced the dao. They understood the principle of balance, of yin and yang, as represented by the transformation of the energies of the universe. Thus they formulated practices...*
> *to promote the flow of qi and...to help maintain and harmonize themselves with the universe. They ate a balanced diet at regular times, arose and retired at regular hours, avoided overstressing their bodies and minds, and refrained from overindulgence of all*

kinds. They maintained well-being of body and mind. Thus it is not surprising that they lived to over one hundred years.

These days, people have changed their way of life. They drink wine as though it were water, indulge excessively in destructive activities, drain their essence, and deplete their qi. They do not know the secret of conserving their energy and vitality. Seeking emotional excitement and momentary pleasures, people disregard the natural rhythm and order of the universe. They fail to regulate their lifestyle and diet, and sleep improperly. So it is not surprising that they look old at fifty and die soon after. (Robinson 2007, p. 85)

Significant contemporary scientific evidence exists supporting this wisdom regarding the efficacy and value of the four pillars of self-care. When you're ready to learn more, you'll find many superb books and other resources that describe the theory and practice of various aspects of these core pillars. (See Resources, at the end of the book, for some recommended texts.)

Pillar 1: Nutrition—You Are What You Eat

It's obvious, yet easily overlooked, that what we eat becomes part of our bodies. It is also well-known that our bodies are in a constant state of flux—our cells are continually turning over and our very substance replacing itself with new ingredients. Those building blocks come from what we ingest, and the primary source of that ingestion is the food we eat. There can be no argument that you are what you eat, so watch what you eat and know what is in it—soon it will be you!

It is not the mission of *Deep Medicine* to recommend one particular diet or approach to eating. However, here are some general guidelines for ensuring that the food you eat is health creating, not health negating:

❀ Regardless of your present diet of choice, notice the size of your portions. As a general rule of thumb, an appropriate portion is about the size of your fist.

- Calories do count! Low-fat and nonfat foods still have calories. And contrary to the popular joke, breaking cookies in half, eating ice cream out of the container, or eating standing up (or when nobody can see you) does not lower the number of calories you consume.

- Balance your intake of carbohydrates, protein, and fat. The once popular high-carbohydrate, low-fat, low-protein approach to weight control may leave you hungry sooner and may not be a healthful choice for you. The well-known high-protein, high-fat diet option has staunch proponents but demonstrates high recidivism (that is, the lost weight is regained). Don't allow yourself to be drawn uncritically to the diet of the moment; we are all individuals, and it's important to figure out what works best for you. What is important is consuming high-quality carbohydrates, fats, and proteins in balanced proportions. This means emphasizing whole grains and complex carbohydrates rather than simple sugars, unsaturated vegetable oils rather than animal-based saturated fats, and varied low-fat sources of protein.

- Seek fresh, locally grown, certified organic fruit and vegetables and emphasize them in your daily menus. A colorful diet is generally a healthful diet. With fruits and vegetables, the fist-sized portion guideline can often be safely exceeded, so enjoy that big bowl of salad! And yes, an apple a day can help keep the doctor away.

- The terms "natural" and "organic" deserve special mention. Products with either of these designations are not universally healthful. Read labels carefully and be alert for added sugars, salt, and unhealthful fats, such as trans fats or lard. In most states, the term "organic" can be used only when particular criteria are met, but the word "natural" is used more loosely. Mercury, hemlock, arsenic, cyanide, poisonous mushrooms, and radioactivity are all natural—and all can be hazardous to your health. And allergic reactions, cross-reactions, or side effects can occur with organic products, just as with conventional products.

🌿 Stay well hydrated. The advice to drink eight glasses of water each day may be excessive for many, but the goal of adequate hydration is sound. Water makes up a large percentage of your body's content and needs to be replenished. It may sound like conflicting advice, but to avoid dehydration, drink before you feel thirsty and also trust your body to tell you when it's thirsty. If drinking eight glasses of water per day leads to excessive trips to the bathroom and you notice your urine is clear, you may be drinking too much. Seek to maintain a light yellow color to your urine. Neither pale, clear urine nor deeply colored, concentrated urine indicates a good balance point.

🌿 Don't forget your need for fiber. Opt for whole grains for the health of your digestive system and for better nutrition.

🌿 Use multiple protein sources, emphasizing soy, fish, low-fat poultry, and nonfat dairy products.

🌿 Stay alert and current regarding reports of contamination, such as mercury in fish, toxins in plastic bottles, and bacteria in raw or improperly cooked foods. When possible, choose local, seasonal, organic items, and for the health of the planet, purchase in bulk or buy foods in nontoxic and reusable packaging.

🌿 Make olive oil your oil of choice, and be sure to consume omega-3 fatty acids, which are good for reducing potential cardiac risk factors. Omega-3s are found in oily fish, such as salmon and sardines, as well as in canola, flaxseed, and walnut oils, and to a lesser degree in soy oil.

🌿 Garlic and ginger are tasty, beneficial ingredients. Garlic is a tonic for the cardiovascular system, reducing cholesterol and triglyceride levels, clumping of platelets, and blood pressure. It also fortifies the immune system and has antibacterial and antifungal effects. Ginger is good for the digestive system and also has anti-inflammatory properties, which can help reduce aches and pains. Turmeric, another popular seasoning, also has anti-inflammatory properties.

🌿 Small quantities of alcohol are acceptable. Remember, however, that alcohol has a high calorie content and little nutritive or medicinal value, the antioxidants in red wine notwithstanding.

🌿 Minimize your consumption of caffeine.

🌿 Minimize your consumption of sweets. Although they taste good and may have emotional appeal, they usually offer only empty calories. Avoid foods and beverages with added sugar and high fructose corn syrup. Chocolate lovers, don't despair. This esteemed food is a valuable source of antioxidants. But do seek out organic, minimally sweetened, dark chocolate. Using cinnamon is a healthful and flavorful substitute for adding more sugar.

🌿 Choose foods with a high nutritional content. These so-called superfoods include avocados, blueberries, broccoli, edamame, flaxseeds, garlic, hemp seeds, kale, kiwi, lentils, nuts, quinoa, salmon (wild), sardines, spinach, tomatoes, turmeric, and yogurt (preferably unsweetened Greek yogurt).

🌿 Keep in mind that how you eat may be as important as what you eat. Prepare your food with respect.

🌿 Turn off the television, light a candle, say grace, eat slowly, and stop eating before you feel full.

As part of your nutritional self-assessment, repeatedly ask yourself what, when, where, how, and even why you are eating. The ayurveda system of health emphasizes bodily constitution types in its approach to nutrition and health and weight management. An individualized approach of this type may be extremely valuable when other, more familiar programs have proved unsuccessful or are unappealing.

Useful resources on nutrition and diet include *The Omega Diet*, by Artemis P. Simopoulos, MD, and Jo Robinson; *Eat More, Weigh Less*, by Dr. Dean Ornish; *The Zone*, by Barry Sears with Bill Lawren; *Eating Well for Optimum Health*, by Andrew Weil, MD; *The Healing Secrets of Food*, by Deborah Kesten; and *Inner Beauty*, by Reenita Malhotra Hora. (For more complete information on these texts, see Resources, at the end of the book.)

Supplements

Vitamins, minerals, and other supplements are valuable as part of a daily health program, but they are supplements, not substitutes for good food. Furthermore, just because small amounts of something are beneficial does not mean that more is better. Excessive use of supplements can cause side effects, overdose, and toxicity, so use over-the-counter products with care. Although vitamins derived from your daily food and beverage intake are almost always more beneficial than a pill, commercially available supplements are useful additions to a health-creating diet. A busy lifestyle, missed meals, environmental contaminants, and daily stressors all are reasons that supplements are potentially valuable as part of a well-rounded nutrition plan.

Be sure to include antioxidants in your supplements—vitamins A (in the form of beta-carotene), C, and E. They help to reduce breakdown at a cellular level and may aid resistance to disease and support longevity. A daily low-dose aspirin may be a valuable addition because of its cardiovascular and anti-inflammatory effects. However, be sure your doctors, especially any surgeons, know you're taking aspirin, because it prolongs bleeding and inhibits clot formation (as do high doses of vitamin E, ginkgo biloba, and several other herbs). The minerals iron, potassium, chromium, calcium, magnesium, selenium, and zinc may be worth supplementing, but keep in mind that any supplement program must be individualized. For example, iron supplementation generally isn't recommended for older men, but is for menstruating women.

You can learn more about other supplements and products that might be useful additions to your wellness program at a library or health food store, on the Internet, or through your favorite practitioner. Here are some examples of specific supplements that can be useful for specific conditions:

- Echinacea and goldenseal root for upper respiratory illness
- Saint-John's-wort taken orally for mild depression and used topically in oil to relieve skin irritation
- Arnica for injuries, swelling, and bruises
- Ginseng as a general tonic
- Ginkgo for circulation and mental alertness
- Aloe vera for burns, dermatitis, and dry skin
- Chamomile as a tea or bath for its sedative properties
- Glucosamine sulfate, chondroitin sulfate, and MSM (methylsulfonylmethane) for arthritis and joint problems

Recommendations regarding supplements and their dosages change frequently as new information becomes available. For example, neurotransmitters, alpha-lipoic acid, L-acetyl carnitine, glutamine, vitamin D, and coenzyme Q10, and a dizzying array of phytochemicals are receiving considerable attention, and new discoveries appear regularly. So avoid the temptation to lock into a particular protocol. Keep your knowledge base current, and do what doctors do: Modify your practices as new information becomes available. A good way to stay current is to subscribe to a wellness newsletter from a reputable source, such as the University of California School of Public Health, *Consumer Reports*, the Mayo Clinic, the Johns Hopkins School of Medicine, or Dr. Andrew Weil.

Also remember that nourishment comes from sources other than those you eat and drink. You ingest via your breath, thoughts, emotions, and senses, so take care to nourish yourself mindfully in all of these domains as well.

Within our current knowledge base, good references regarding diet, supplements, and general well-being include books in the series You, the Owners Manual, by Drs. Mehmet Oz and Michael Roizen; *Optimal Wellness*, by Ralph Golan, MD; *Encyclopedia of Natural Medicine*, by Michael Murray, ND, and Joseph Pizzorno, ND; *Prescription for Nutritional Healing*, by James and Phyllis Balch; and *A Clinician's Guide to Holistic Medicine*, by Robert A. Anderson, MD.

Pillar 2: Physical Activity—Move It or Lose It

The body is your home for your adventure on Earth. You must treat it with honor and respect or you'll find yourself without a place to live. As the vehicle for your life's journey, your body must be well maintained so that you can live your innermost dreams and manifest your gifts and talents in the world.

Physical activity may be the most important thing you can do for your well-being. If there is anything that might be considered a fountain of youth, exercise would probably come the closest. Your body wants to be used, not saved. Exercise is a powerful force in the management of weight, diabetes, cardiovascular health, depression, stress, immune system function, and aging. In fact, for sustainable, long-term weight management, your dietary practices must be paired with exercise.

The benefits of exercise are most dramatic when comparing the well-being of the couch potato and the walker, not the walker and the marathon runner. In other words, you don't have to spend endless hours at the gym to achieve results. Walking, climbing stairs, household activities like vacuuming, and social activities like dancing count, too. Don't forget to stretch and rest, or exercise might create as many problems as it helps.

Your exercise program needs to include activities that support balance and flexibility, as well as cardiovascular fitness, breathing, and strength training (resistance training is especially recommended for women at menopause). Practices such as yoga, tai chi, and qigong (and others, like Feldenkrais and Pilates) are especially beneficial, since they incorporate the full spectrum of balancing, stretching, and strengthening activities, along with meditative and breathing exercises.

And don't neglect your posture. The alignment of your body while both standing and sitting is critical to full breathing, provides adequate space for your abdominal organs, allows proper movement of your arms and legs, and minimizes musculoskeletal discomfort. Keep in mind that healthy posture can help prevent many of the deformities of aging, such as rounding of the shoulders, collapse of the chest, loss of the lumbar curve, and forward protrusion of the neck and head, along with their associated pain and limitations.

Breath and breathing link us to life. We take our first breath at birth and our last at our death. Learning to breathe properly is an important aspect of well-being. All too often, people breathe primarily into the chest. Abdominal or belly breathing allows for deeper breathing, better exchange of the gases essential for life, and relaxation. This is because the diaphragm—the muscle between the abdomen and chest—descends toward the belly, filling the lungs more deeply. On exhalation, the belly falls back toward the spine as the diaphragm rises and the lungs empty. When you're breathing naturally, a slight pause occurs after each inhalation and exhalation. Consciously lengthening your exhalation in relationship to your inhalation will slow your breathing and enhance relaxation. As you become more aware of and practiced at the mechanics of good breath work, and as you breathe more consciously and intentionally, your breathing will become more effective and efficient, as will your periods of exercise and relaxation.

A moderate daily dose of exercise is safer and more beneficial than infrequent extended bouts. Weekend warriors take note: Thirty to sixty minutes five times a week is a common recommendation. As little exercise as ten minutes three times per day can provide that thirty minutes and make a significant difference for your well-being. You don't have to go to the gym, health club, or swimming pool or have a room full of equipment at home to achieve this goal. Climbing the stairs at work, taking a walk after dinner, or using your own body as an exercise device (as in push-ups, sit-ups, and so on) will be more effective than sophisticated exercise equipment or classes you have access to but don't use.

Variety is the spice of life when it comes to exercise. A varied program is less likely to become boring and therefore more likely to become an ongoing part of your daily life. Not only is it okay for your exercise program to be fun, it is mandatory for a sustainable plan. Different times of day have different advantages, and we all have our preferences. What's most important is that you actually commit to an exercise program, devise one that fits your needs, and then make the time to exercise. The best exercise is the one you do! Depending on your age and the state of your health, you may need to consult with your doctor first or work with a teacher or trainer.

Don't forget that your brain and mind require exercise, too. Use your mind, whether in the form of doing puzzles, philosophizing, brushing your teeth with your nondominant hand, or not sitting at the same place at the dining room table for every meal. These changes of habit stimulate the brain and nervous system. Thus they may foster mental agility and lessen the risk of dementia. Your brain likes to practice things it enjoys and finds interesting. Furthermore, it remembers what it practices repeatedly, and practice and memory are essential components of creating good habits.

To balance your physical activity and exercise, you need adequate rest and sleep. Seven to nine hours of sleep are usually recommended. Inadequate sleep is cumulative and leads to chronic sleep deprivation, which is a recognized health hazard. If the amount and patterns of your sleep are compromised, you are putting your well-being at risk and may need to seek expert help. Try to go to sleep at a consistent time most nights. Avoid stimulants of all sorts before retiring; this includes late-night news shows, intense conversations or arguments, large meals, and vigorous exercise. Never underestimate the value of a good night's sleep and even a nap.

Useful resources in regard to exercise and fitness include *Body, Mind, and Spirit: The Mind-Body Guide to Lifelong Fitness and Your Personal Best*, by John Douillard; *Wellness Medicine*, by Robert A.

Anderson, MD; *Women's Bodies, Women's Wisdom*, by Christiane Northrup, MD; *The Wellness Guide to Lifelong Fitness*, by Timothy White; and *Ultra-Longevity*, by Mark Liponis, MD.

Pillar 3: Relationship and Community—When Two or More Are Gathered

True independence is a myth. Social isolation is a risk factor for heart disease as significant as smoking, and a supportive community is a powerful healing force. There are both power and intelligence of great profundity in the creation of community.

Relationship is an essential part of the healing journey and of all healing encounters. A certain amount of time spent with others is necessary for health. Yet the most important relationship of all is with yourself. From that, we build other relationships, from the intimate sphere to groups, then the natural world, and ultimately the realm of the sacred. The recognition that, ultimately, we are all interconnected and interdependent is a vital part of deep medicine, as is the development of effective communication skills and practices.

Tips for Developing Healthy Relationships

Make time to be with others on a one-to-one basis and in groups. Move your relational work beyond your inner circle of family and friends. True compassion and caring for others must not be limited to our intimates; it must extend to all our relations and to the greater good. Intergenerational relationships are highly valuable. Visit with elders; they have much to teach us that our youth-oriented culture disregards. Enjoy the company of children; they need the guidance, and we need the fun. Don't overlook the importance of walking your dog or stroking your cat; interspecies relationships are meaningful, too.

Practice direct communication in your intimate and group relationships. Make amends, forgive indiscretions, and avoid gossip. Don't harbor resentments until they boil into something scalding and become very hurtful. When questions arise, confusion is apparent, or feelings are hurt, practice early check-ins to allow for clarification, apology, and rectification. This will help avoid further injury and create the context for healing.

Communication skills are essential to healthy relationships. There is probably no knowledge base more resonant or skill set more valuable than the fundamentals of direct, honest, timely communications. Always remember that good communication isn't just about the words you use. Body language and tonality often communicate more than words. That is why in-person communication is the most complete, and why misunderstandings may occur over the phone or via the written word, especially via e-mail, where hints from body language and tone can't help convey the message. Check in frequently for clarification if you have doubts about what was said, what you heard, or what happened. Don't make assumptions or speculate; ask for confirmation or repeat back what you think you heard. Be clear and make it clear how you feel and how you have interpreted what others communicate.

Valuable learning tools for communications include audio programs by Patrick O'Neill of Toronto, Canada, entitled *Extraordinary Conversations*. Also highly recommended are the books, CDs, and tapes of Angeles Arrien; *Difficult Conversations: How to Discuss What Matters Most*, by Douglas Stone, Bruce Patton, and Sheila Heen; *Nonviolent Communication: A Language of Life*, by Marshall Rosenberg; and *Crucial Conversations: Tools for Talking When Stakes Are High*, by Kerry Patterson, Joseph Grenny, Ron McMillan, and Al Switzler.

Honoring Your Relationship with Nature

When it comes to regulating the rhythm of our lives in a health-creating way, a relationship to nature and its cycles can be a more meaningful timekeeper than our wristwatches, electronic calendars, and alarm clocks. Nature's usual pace is medium to slow. High-speed activities, such as chasing prey, last only for brief periods of time. In contrast, the usual pace in our culture is fast to overdrive. One of the most rejuvenating aspects of my vacations is the chance to allow my body to function in accordance with its own internal rhythm, without external timekeeping aids. A health-creating holiday is one where I get up when I'm through sleeping, eat when I feel hungry, and follow a schedule based on internal requirements rather than external demands.

Time in natural settings allows us to reestablish or strengthen our relationship with Mother Nature and her rhythms. It allows us to reacquaint ourselves with aspects of our being that may go unvisited during our usual day-to-day life. The wilderness experience is conducive to giving gratitude, seeking guidance, acknowledging, connecting, and regaining perspective. It provides the opportunity for ritual and ceremony, two essential ingredients for reverent, mindful, healthy living. Walking in the woods, climbing a mountain, swimming in the ocean, napping on a beach, working in the garden, watching a sunrise or sunset, listening to a babbling brook, feeling the dew on your bare feet or the wind in your face are all experiences that refresh the spirit, reconnect us to natural rhythms, and create openings for growth and healing.

Make time to be in nature on a daily basis, whether alone or with others, even if only to take a walk around the block.

Relating Through Play

Ancient humans didn't spend all their time hunting, gathering, and seeking shelter. They also devoted a certain amount of time to sitting around the fire, dancing, and storytelling. They spent a good bit more time in leisure activities and relating to each other and the world around them than we do—even with our plethora of so-called labor-saving and time-saving devices.

Work dominates contemporary life. We work not only to provide our material needs, but to be of service and to define our self-image and sense of worth, purpose, and meaning. However, we are neither our accomplishments nor our mistakes, and we aren't "wasting time" when we are at play or at rest, particularly when those activities allow us to deepen our connections with others.

Adjusting your concept of productive time to include play is essential. Playtime needs to be nourishing, not mind deadening (such as watching more television) or thrill seeking (the adventure-junkie syndrome). To balance your relationship to work with sufficient rest and recreation, you need to spend some of your time nurturing your inner needs and recharging your batteries, not competing in contexts where performance or approval is the goal. The work-rest dynamic is another example of wholeness and health requiring a balance between doing and being. Taking breaks at work, eating lunch someplace other than at your desk, or going outside if you work inside can replenish your energy. Listening to music, singing, or even something as simple as rocking in a rocking chair can contribute to positive emotions and ease anxiousness, fatigue, and insecurity.

Pillar 4: Contemplation and Solitude— Awakening Your Inner Healer

Wholeness is an expression of health. Practices that connect our outer and inner landscapes foster wholeness and lead us to where we can harness the source of our healing power. The deep inner dimension of existence and the vast expanse and unseen presence that surround our physical bodies cannot be discounted in any quest for health and healing. Any practice that helps connect us to our true inner selves can be a health-creating or healing endeavor. While many practices begin in classes and with explicit physical instructions related to body placement and movement, they ultimately become personal and spiritual experiences. Expanded or more focused applications of such practices as a regular exercise program, the formal practice of yoga or tai chi, or a defined time for philosophic readings, contemplation, meditation, or prayer are all opportunities for solitude and contemplation. These moments can be used for relaxation, giving thanks, setting intention, and reverence for all that contributes to making up our lives.

Early on in your practice, these brief moments of contemplative experience may create a desire to spend more time in such activities, opening the door to further personal exploration and growth. From here you will be led to teachers, mentors, and even communities that will support your seeking as you explore your paths to awareness, health, and healing.

The Four Practices

Four practices common among many cultures—slowing down, getting quiet, paying attention, and going inward—carry us toward our inner landscape, allowing us to contact our true selves and awaken our inner healing power. These four practices lead to the development of self-awareness and create the possibility of seeing our true essence, free of roles, titles, expectations, and judgments.

Slowing down. You can't access your inner wisdom while living in the fast lane, multitasking, skipping breakfast, and rushing to your next obligation.

Getting quiet. The surrounding din of ever-present telephones, television, Internet, personal music, and frequent interactions and interruptions brings constant noise to our lives. You must find a patch of quiet to access your inner landscape and healing wisdom.

Paying attention. We are easily distracted and diverted in the course of our daily lives. To access the wisdom available within, you have to pay attention and tune in to the channel that's relevant in the present moment.

Going inward. Our attention, gaze, and hearing are usually directed outward, toward where we think we're going. Looking to the external world is the realm of doing. Exploring the inner world brings us to the realm of being. Always remember, we are human *beings*, not just human *doings*. Both spheres, being and doing, must come together to fully foster wholeness and health. To harvest the lessons of your inner world, you must direct your attention inward through practices such as taking a walk on a labyrinth, meditating, praying, spending a quiet day alone, or engaging in a spiritual practice that calls to you. Such practices can help you connect with your inner purpose and meaning and your life's passion and dream. Then it becomes possible to begin to align your inner wisdom with your active work toward health, healing, and service to yourself and others.

Your inner world has a powerful impact and is inseparable from your outer world. The four practices, like the four pillars, will guide you to places of self-discovery. This is where your self-identity and creative purpose are formed upon the landscape of faith and fear, worry and wishes, dreams and disappointments, joy and sadness, intuition and coincidence, grief and belief, and inspiration and imagination. You won't find this territory on a physical map, but it is nonetheless real. This hidden sphere has many names: the individual soul, the realm of spirit, mystery, the infinite, and numerous others. Whatever its name, you will experience it via inner stillness and through awe, being, and becoming. John O'Donohue put it well in his book *Anam Cara: Spiritual Wisdom from the Celtic World* (1998, p. xvi):

> *If we become addicted to the external, our interiority will haunt us. We will become hungry with a hunger no image, person, or deed can still. To be wholesome, we must remain truthful to our vulnerable complexity. In order to keep our balance, we need to hold the interior and exterior, visible and invisible, known and unknown, temporal and eternal, ancient and new, together. No one else can undertake this task for you. You are the one and the only threshold of an inner world. This wholesomeness is holiness. To be holy is to be natural, to befriend the worlds that come to balance in you. Behind the facade of image and distraction, each person is...an inner artist who carries and shapes a unique world.*

In times of personal and global tension, fear, despair, and longing, you must attend to your inner life as carefully as your outer life. There are many routes to accessing your inner dimension, but they share the overarching principle that silence is golden. Time for quiet and solitude is absolutely necessary in your self-care program and is at the heart of stress management. Just as the foods you eat provide nutrients and energy for your physical being, slowing down and finding quiet are the sources of nourishment for your inner life. This is part of the balance that health is, a corollary to necessary movement. Reading the classics and works of ancient wisdom can provide respite and insight. Daily exposure to words of wisdom is a needed antidote to the barrage of television infotainment and the heavy overstimulation that modern communication provides our senses.

Now that you understand the philosophy behind the four practices, and the healing power inherent in them, let's take a look at some ways and places to apply them.

Inner Wisdom

Each of us needs to escape the incessant noise that surrounds us—everyday business, social chatter, mass media—to create the opening to connect with our inner wisdom. This is where deep learning takes place. It is our well of inner wisdom that informs us of our life's dream and steadily guides us toward it. As you begin to silence the surrounding clamor and lessen the distractions that keep you from your vital inner work, you will better hear the inner messages that can guide your choices on your healing path.

Insight meditation teacher Jack Kornfield (1993) shares a story about how to access your inner knowing when you find yourself in a difficult situation—a situation that calls for more wisdom than you can access at the time. Imagine you hear a knock on the door and you open it. There stands _____ (fill in the blank with the guide you need: Jesus, Buddha, Mother Teresa, Gandhi, or whomever). Let this guide trade places with you for a moment, taking your role in the situation. Your guide will advise you about what to do next.

As you fill yourself with the way you imagine your guide would handle the knotty situation, you realize you carry much more potential for wisdom than you usually realize. My older son, when confronted with a problem beyond his skill in Little League baseball, often conjured advice from the baseball sages of days gone by, wondering, "What would Babe Ruth do at a time like this?" Consider a problem you are working on at the present time and try it for yourself.

Finding Time

Exactly what you do with the solitude you create is less important than making the time for it. This time is never wasted. It is as important as mealtime. It is best not to dilute it by doing anything else, including vigorous exercise (though exercise can help free and empty the mind and provide a wonderful but different opportunity for clear internal dialogues and expression).

Whether you sit, stand, lie, or walk; recite an affirmation or mantra; chant, pray, or count your breaths; open or close your eyes; do yoga, meditate, or play music—the essential thing is to quiet your mind and be fully in the moment. Stay with the peace and calm of the present. Don't fight the thoughts that will inevitably show up; just let them pass. Don't resist the sounds you hear; just let them be. Don't fight the restlessness you feel; just be with it.

Start by keeping a daily appointment with yourself to be alone and slow down, get quiet, pay attention, and go inward. Initially, make your appointment as short as necessary to ensure you will do it. Then gradually increase your time commitment. Practice, persevere, and continue making the effort. You will be rewarded by the clarity these practices bring you, which will actually give you extra time in the long run. Disconnect these practices from any particular goal and do them for their own intrinsic worth—your full awareness. Whether you have five minutes or sixty minutes, start with whatever time you have.

You can experience the effects of these practices—even in *one minute*. These "magic moments" of silence, breath awareness, focused attention, relaxation, and the like can give you a taste of the benefits of a longer practice, such as twenty minutes of meditation or sixty to ninety minutes of yoga.

It Only Takes a Minute: The Deep Minute

The use of frequent deep minutes provides an entry point to changing your mind one minute at a time. This brief time of slowing down and getting quiet provides an opening for you to experience awareness, appreciation, acknowledgment of self and others, calmness, gratitude, clarity, forgiveness, intention, insight, anger management, relaxation, stress reduction, creative problem solving, deep listening, inspiration, intuition, creativity, or imagination. In the deep minute, you begin to practice new behaviors that are truly health creating, sustainable, and transformative.

I first began using the practice of the deep minute many years ago when I would lecture to young doctors in surgical training. These lectures usually occurred at the end of a long and busy day. Many of the young surgeons had worked ten to twelve hours without time to rest or eat. Before beginning the formal lecture for which we were scheduled, we would share a deep minute—literally sixty seconds of quiet contemplation to help all of us arrive at the present moment together and release what had come before and what was yet to come in our busy day. For some the minute seemed very short, and for others it felt much longer than just sixty seconds. For most of us, it was the longest period of repose we had enjoyed during the day. During those deep minutes, it was apparent how powerful this simple technique could be for our personal and collective sense of well-being.

Entering a deep minute involves simply taking the time in the course of a busy day to pause, bring attention to whatever you wish, and quietly allow an opening for a mindful break in ongoing events. It can be done at your desk, on the job, alone, or in a group, with eyes open or closed, and with or without a mantra, chanting, or the counting of your breath. All that is necessary is your full attention. In the process, you will gain equanimity, and foster longer periods of nonreactive balance in your daily life. This is a small, early step toward an enduring wisdom practice. You can engage in a deep minute anytime, anyplace, and for any reason you wish. All you need to do is do it!

The Deep Minute

To enter a deep minute, sit upright in a chair or on the floor on a pillow or meditation bolster if you choose. If on a bolster on the floor, sit cross-legged or on your heels with your knees bent and your shins and the top of your feet on a blanket or mat. If on a chair and it is comfortable and possible for you, align yourself so that your ears are over your shoulders (that is, your head is not jutting forward), your shoulders over your hips, your knees over your ankles, and your feet flat on the floor, parallel and pointing straight ahead. Elevate your sternum (breastbone) and lower ribs, soften your belly, relax your shoulders away from your ears, allow your hands to rest comfortably on your thighs with palms up or down, cupped on top of each other or with your fingertips lightly touching.

Breathe through your nose deeply, slowly, and without force or strain. Allow your breath to breathe you. There is great intelligence in our bodies. Our innate cellular wisdom knows how to keep our breathing, heartbeat, digestion, and myriad other bodily actions going without our being consciously aware of or in volitional control of these processes. Close your eyes gently or softly defocus them, looking slightly downward, and relax your jaw. Then simply sit quietly for a minute. As your practice with the deep minute matures, you will probably choose to spend more than just one minute in this restful state. Even a single minute, however, can begin to connect you with your inner world of being.

The Payoff

Every minute is a new creative experience, never lived before, never to be lived again. Every moment that we enter with full awareness is a true gift and a practice of being present and mindful of what actually is (the present)—not what was (the past) or what might be (the future). Living in the moment, minute by minute, is a wisdom practice. Since it is your practice, it cannot be judged or compared to anyone else's. But you must be present to win! This practice cannot be replaced by exercise or sleep; it is about being fully awake—fully present, mindfully aware in the moment—and quiet.

As you practice, you will notice your thought processes settling like mud settles when agitated water becomes still. You will begin to gain awareness of your bodily sensations and emotions—your visceral responses to what happens around you. You will be more in touch with yourself and your environment. Can you be patient and wait for the mud to settle and the water to clear? If you can, you will note your pulse rate slowing, your breathing slowing and deepening, and your body releasing the tension it holds.

The practices taught in meditation classes, stress reduction centers, behavior modification programs, yoga classes, and the like provide technical instruction in quieting the mind. This is useful, but you must spread this awareness into your day-to-day life, rather than relegating it to once a week during group or class time.

Mindfulness means being fully present, in a nonjudgmental way, with whatever you are doing: sitting, jogging, eating, washing the dishes, cleaning up a mess, talking with a friend, negotiating a deal, listening to a sales pitch, driving a car, or even working at your job. These activities can all be done mindfully, with your full attention. Even when you are remembering the lessons of the past or planning for the future, do it from the context of the present: don't let planning or remembering distract you from your present reality, but rather, experience these processes actively in the moment you are consciously living as you do them.

Daily Blessings

Helen Keller said, "I long to accomplish a great and noble task, but it is my chief duty to accomplish small tasks as if they were great and noble." The creation of health, and harnessing the sources of your healing power, may at times seem overwhelming—a great and noble task, but perhaps unattainable. It is the small steps done mindfully that get you there. During the course of your daily life, you have many opportunities to connect your personal life to the bigger picture. By slowing down and doing something in a meaningful way, you change your relationship to time, creating sacred time and space as you experience your connection and interplay with all around you. The simplest acts—retiring in the evening, arising in the morning, preparing or eating a meal, taking a shower—can give you the opportunity to pause, set your intention, and give thanks. In so doing, activities that otherwise might seem mundane are transformed into sacred, purposeful, and meaningful actions.

Doing something purposefully can turn it into a personal ritual that fosters your well-being by helping you slow down and carve out a quiet space, allowing you to go inward to honor, give gratitude, pray, or reflect. This is another definition of mindfulness: doing whatever it is you are doing with attention to the task and intention to create real purpose, meaning, or value for the task. Furthermore, mindful practice of daily activities encourages responsibility for our actions.

For example, contemplating a seed as you plant it can connect you with the potential inherent in even the smallest of things. Approaching a meal mindfully can connect you with the incredible network that brought the food to your table, starting with the earth, sun, and water. You can imagine the farmer, the fieldworker, and the baker of the bread. Then there are their families, who support them in their work, and those who transport, process, and sell the food, and on and on. How incredibly interconnected our lives are. Even if you raised the produce for your salad in your own garden, the connections and relationships are similarly extensive.

When you relate to your daily activities with this kind of clear attention, from exercise to eating to working and playing, you will experience the health benefits that come with mindful living. You'll exercise more often because it makes you feel better. Your diet and eating practices will shift as you consider more than just calories and pounds, engaging questions of when and why you eat. Through frequent, conscious self-assessment, you become intimate with your own body and its functions. From this awareness, your capacity to be intimate with others will also benefit.

As you become familiar with your inner landscape, you will begin to create your own personal rituals. For example, you may choose to include a period of silence as part of your morning routine. Or perhaps you'll simply take a moment or two at the start of your day to breathe quietly and naturally to provide grounding relaxation and add a sense of sacredness to the day.

Some people find it valuable to create a small altar somewhere in their home—a place where ancestors, friends, and family members can be remembered and honored or where milestones can be recalled with small mementos. Visiting your altar as part of a morning routine can provide a time and place to pray for others who are ill or in need of guidance, and to speak the names of loved ones to be remembered.

In the transformative moment of silence that you experience at your personal altar, you can also consider what lies ahead in the coming day and what resources or strengths will serve you best. Perhaps you need flexibility, a sense of humor, or patience. Whatever it might be, you can ask for help and prepare yourself for what is to come. Yet even as you do this, recognize that the agenda and game plan you have in mind may not be exactly what happens, or what the universe, mystery, or the divine has on tap for you.

Always be open to what might show up, not just what you expect or hope for. Oftentimes, expectations set you up for failure, unhappiness, or disappointment. It's worthwhile to be aware of the potential for things not going as you expect. Maintain an attitude of curiosity and a sense of humor. Give everything you do your full attention and best effort, then accept the outcome with interest and curiosity and be prepared to correct your course as necessary.

Excellent references regarding the inner landscape, in addition to John O'Donohue's *Anam Cara*, include *Sabbath: Restoring the Sacred Rhythm of Rest*, by Wayne Muller; *The Miracle of Mindfulness*, by Thich Nhat Hanh; *Wherever You Go, There You Are*, by Jon Kabat-Zinn; *A Path with Heart*, by Jack Kornfield; *Don't Just Do Something, Sit There*, by Sylvia Boorstein; *Walking a Sacred Path*, by Lauren Artress; and *The Power of Now*, by Eckhart Tolle.

Cultivating New Sources of Wisdom

Not long ago I had the privilege of attending a retreat as part of the transformative work done by the Institute of Noetic Sciences in Petaluma, California. One of the exercises involved taking time in silence on the beautiful rolling hills that surround its campus. We were sent out onto the land with a ceremony that included drumming and using one of the oldest tools of indigenous cultures, the rattle. We were given several questions to consider and advised to be alert and attentive to the signs that the land might present to us to help us with the questions we were contemplating.

I set off with lofty expectations. What powerful allies might make themselves visible to me? What wisdom would the call of Brother

Raven or the spirit of native peoples who previously walked this land reveal? As I began my meditative walk, I was drawn to a fallen, partially uprooted tree. While some branches were dead or dying, others were clearly green and robust. I was moved to notice that we are subject to forces that can significantly disrupt our roots and direction. Some parts of us die along the way even as others continue to grow. We have different uses at different times. But I felt this wasn't the place for me to stop.

I carried on farther until I came to a fence line. The fence called me to respect the limits and boundaries of the collective, myself, and others. As I climbed higher on the hillside, I could hear the noise from the freeway not far from the entrance to the wooded enclave. Slightly higher on the hill, I could look down and into the distance and see the dense line of cars on the highway—a river of machinery flowing slowly toward San Francisco. I imagined the stress the slow traffic was causing and could almost hear the crackle of engaged cell phones and feel the sense of urgency of the people trapped in that gnarled, phlegmatic, bumper-to-bumper crawl. "Leave the collective trance. Don't be confined by what seems to be so important—look further," was the message for me.

I continued my silent wandering. As I walked, I waited for a vision more profound than the freeway, a symbol more remarkable than the fence or the fallen tree, a helping ally more dignified than a lizard sunning on a dull, flat rock. Where was the soaring raven, the elusive mountain lion?

I moved on up the hill toward the summit, expectations ablaze. When I crested the top and could see a 360-degree panorama, I was shocked to behold a large, abandoned tractor tire. How disappointing! Others had been here before, and this was not an artifact to be cherished—or was it? Amused, I sat down on the large, black remnant of another's previous visit to my chosen destination. As I surveyed the hilltop, I noticed that there was a message for me encoded on my perch: "Goodyear," it read. A *good year*—how prophetic. My curiosity aroused, I wondered what else the circular oracle might reveal. I swept its dusty surface and was rewarded as more advice appeared. While a good year was prominently predicted, some cautions were also noted: "Failure may be due to misapplication, improper inflation (over- or underinflation), overloading, excessive speed, and improper mounting."

What germane and powerful wisdom! And how different its source than my romantic expectations. Isn't it interesting when and where we can find wisdom if we are open to seeing and hearing it? As the distant drumbeat beckoned me to return to the circle of my colleagues, where we would share our journeys, I descended the hill once again, surprised and moved by the healing wisdom I had found in such a seemingly mundane and unlikely source.

KNOW YOUR SELF, HEAL YOURSELF

Working with the pillars and practices described in this chapter can help you connect your inner aspirations and dreams with health-creating external actions. Many times the steps toward fulfilling your dreams or responding to your calling will be small, and they may be challenged or limited by pressures such as familial and financial obligations. However, even small steps can help reduce anxiety and keep you in alignment with your innermost needs and desires. Your task is to discover your unique inner gifts—your medicine—and to bring that medicine into your life. No one can do it for you, and no one can tell you what it should look like. We are all offered the raw material and some rudimentary instructions, but each of us must find the way on our own.

This work of discovering and harnessing the source of your healing power is deep medicine. Medicine for your body, mind, and spirit. It is a lifelong process of continuous learning in which you'll need to correct your course many times. You also need to take time afterward to integrate what you've learned into your daily life. This deep work will reward you with a great wealth of energy for your pursuit of health and healing. What you give up in nonproductive behaviors and the quest for an elusive quick fix will be returned many times over in the sense of well-being that you will achieve along your healing path of authentic self-awareness, self-discovery, and self-expression.

EXERCISES FOR CHAPTER 4: WHERE THE RUBBER HITS THE ROAD

Exercise 1: A Workout for Inner Strength

Many of us spend a great deal of time and money working out: exercising, stretching, and working to shape and tone our bodies. Most of these activities are directed primarily at our outer strength. What about building our inner strength? How do we forge the endurance for inner challenges? How do we develop the flexibility, agility, and strength to deal with the various habits, behaviors, fears, and stresses that trouble us?

We need workouts, exercises, and practices for growing our inner resources as well as our outer, external strengths. Yet we must also stay alert to how these practices can become limitations, addictions, or obstacles—not just tools and aids—if they are misused. Interestingly, we often make choices that ultimately work against developing inner strength. We look for activities that allow us to distract ourselves from the necessary work, numb ourselves to the inner pain, or insulate ourselves from the emptiness or injury we may feel. Material goods, lofty ideals, or so-called spiritual practices in the absence of inner strength building cannot fill us, heal us, or protect us.

Here are some guidelines for building inner strength:

1. Become aware of patterns, behaviors, habits, attitudes, beliefs, thoughts, feelings, and actions that are burdening, obstructing, poisoning, or deterring you.

2. Bring your full attention and consciousness to your highest-priority issues.

3. Determine appropriate action steps to begin remedying those high-priority issues.

4. Maintain curiosity, wonder, and awe at your progress (or lack thereof) and the unfolding of your life. Recall that the most

common place for a major blockage to occur on your path to making health-creating changes is between knowing what you need to do and fully committing to action—that is, between deciding and actually doing.

Consider the four practices for awakening and harnessing your inner healing power: slowing down, getting quiet, paying attention, going inward. How can you apply them to your personal circumstances with specific tools and techniques, such as meditation, yoga, or reconnecting to the spiritual or religious tradition of your upbringing?

Exercise 2: Taking Real Steps

Consider what you have to do to realize your desired health breakthrough, your inner dream or purpose, or your highest-priority goal. Remember that your time is limited and that you have "windows of opportunity" in which to act. Here are some activities to guide you in taking real steps:

🌿 Review the four pillars of self-care (nutrition, physical activity and relaxation, relationship and community, and contemplation and solitude) and consider how each of the pillars is supporting your goals—or not. What do you have to do to change that? Start with small steps.

🌿 In assessing your decision making, consider this riddle: Five frogs are sitting on a log. Four decide to jump off. How many frogs remain sitting on the log? (Hint: Is deciding the same as doing?)

🌿 Do you express your authenticity, your true self? Have you experienced the consequences of not being aware of or expressing what's true for you? Consider this insight by psychologist Abraham Maslow: "If this essential core of the person is denied or suppressed, he gets sick sometimes in obvious ways, sometimes in subtle ways, sometimes immediately, sometimes later" (1999, p. 6). How does this relate to you harnessing the sources of your healing power?

🌢 Consider what a seed gives up to become a sprout. How does that relate to your taking the next necessary step for your well-being?

🌢 Prepare and eat a meal mindfully and gracefully.

🌢 Inventory your personal rituals that transform routine activities into sacred acts.

🌢 Schedule a massage regularly, to help you stay in touch with your physical body.

🌢 Practice saying no to others. It can be a complete sentence: "No."

🌢 Practice saying yes to yourself (be as compassionate with yourself as with others).

🌢 Practice really listening. When someone else is speaking, rather than rehearsing or thinking about what you're going to say next, listen attentively and without being judgmental, then respond in a way that reflects back what you've heard.

🌢 Consider what the saying "Attitude is everything" means in the context of your healing journey.

Exercise 3: Beginning a Daily Practice

Consider starting your day with cultural anthropologist Angeles Arrien's Blessing Way (2005). This simple practice only takes a few minutes:

1. Give gratitude.

2. Set your intention.

3. Perform a life-affirming action in support of your dream, passion, or calling.

This is an easy and powerful way to begin a personal daily practice that will provide an interface between your inner and outer worlds. The possibilities for this practice are endless, and ultimately its form will reflect your unique identity and situation. For example, in the morning you might give gratitude for the dreamtime and for awakening to the rising sun; set an intention to see the spark of the divine in everyone you encounter that day; and support your desire to see your grandchildren by scheduling a day off. Or in the evening, you might give gratitude for returning home safely after a day of work, or say grace over dinner; set an intention to listen more than you talk that evening; and choose to read from a wisdom text, such as the Bhagavad Gita.

Exercise 4: Tips for the Trip

Imagine you encounter a cold, rapidly flowing river along your chosen route. As you look across to the other side and contemplate crossing it, here are some principles to keep in mind:

- Your destination may not be where you thought it was.

- There is no perfect time or place to start.

- The route, and even the rules, are constantly changing.

- You will get cold, wet, and tired and stub your toes (or even lose them).

- You will lose and regain your balance many times.

- Sometimes the way that looks easiest isn't.

- Sometimes the way that looks hardest isn't.

- Proper equipment, instruction, and preparation can aid your progress and success.

- Small steps are okay.

- Stepping backward or sideways is sometimes essential.

- If the crossing is long, you may need to stop and rest. Look ahead for a safe place to do so.

- Although focusing on the specific act at hand is imperative, you must be able to do more than one thing at a time and also remain aware of the big picture.

- Being afraid isn't necessarily bad. Courage doesn't mean being unafraid; it means moving forward in the presence of your fear.

- In spite of your best intentions and efforts, you will encounter circumstances that disrupt your expectations, seeming to hinder your forward progress. However, what seems like a setback may later turn out to be a gift or opportunity.

- You must let go of the need for only rational, objective approaches and trust other ways of knowing, such as intuition, gut feelings, and inner voices.

- When you get to the other side, the tools, equipment, and techniques you used to get there may no longer be useful. Be sure to let go of what you don't need. Today's building blocks may become tomorrow's burden.

CHAPTER 5

Creating Your Own Healing Story

Know thyself.

—Socrates

Everybody is a story.

—Rachel Naomi Remen

Discovering your story is a part of harnessing the source of your healing power. Working with the pillars and practices of self-care described in chapter 4 and making them an integral part of your daily life contributes to the creation of your own healing story. Owning your story honestly, without embellishment, blame, or harsh judgments toward yourself or others, is practicing deep medicine.

Your personal life story is being created in every moment, whether you realize it or not. And the story you tell yourself and others about yourself can either enhance or negate your health and sense of well-being. If you're optimistic and self-assured, your health will be expansive and reflect your positive outlook. By the same token, if you're continually self-critical and negative, your health will suffer accordingly, limiting and compromising all of your relationships, including your primary relationship: the one you have with yourself. Your story, and learning to appreciate who you are through that story, is important to your well-being and to the well-being of others. No one can be healthy and have a healing story without self-respect, self-love, and love for others, qualities that arise out of rigorous self-inquiry and inner work.

Beyond your strictly personal tale, learning the story of your ancestral roots—familial, cultural, and spiritual—links you to your heritage and helps define who you are. Knowing where you came from is an essential part of self-knowledge and is necessary for authenticity. The connection of your story to your own healing path begins with your DNA but is not limited to it. Through the kind of personal exploration that deep medicine exacts, by searching out your roots and the true basis of your behaviors, beliefs, and opinions, you will learn what pushes your buttons, leads you to resist more healthful lifestyle choices, and causes you to react, shut down, collapse, or leave. Through telling your story and listening to others, you come to be known, and you forge the relationships that build trust and deep healing. This process fosters personal transformation, which is the source of lasting social change. This is how the personal, the public, and the planetary become connected. This is how wholeness—the essence of deep medicine—is created: one story at a time

HOW STORIES AFFECT HEALTH

Your story is part of everything you think, feel, say, and do. What you know and believe about yourself, both consciously and unconsciously, has a persistent influence on your health. As you focus on your individual story, you'll undoubtedly see how the hand you've been dealt—

your genetic makeup, your family of origin, your upbringing—impacts your well-being. However, your genes are only one part of that story. As you learned in chapter 4, your lifestyle choices are probably the single most important potentially manageable component in the delicate balance that brings about health and healing. In making these choices, you are shaping how your story unfolds.

While I was a visiting professor at a university medical center, I was introduced to a patient whose situation illustrates how people can be blind to their own story and its influence on their medical status. This patient was a young and generally healthy woman suffering from a severe inflammatory condition around one of her eyes. Her complaints included pain and reduced vision in that eye, along with redness, swelling, and restricted movement of the eye.

She had been extensively questioned and evaluated by the team of physicians responsible for her care. My time with her was short, and my review of the information available showed that the doctors had evaluated her completely only to emerge with essentially normal findings other than those related to her red, inflamed eye. Lacking any definite cause for her problem, such as infection, cancer, or injury, I began to question her further. I asked, "Is there anything going on in your life that you might relate to the onset or progression of your illness?" She thought a moment, then said that nothing unusual was happening.

I probed further, explaining that stress can contribute to many illnesses and asking, "Is there anything happening in your life that you consider stressful?"

"No, everything is going all right. In fact, I was recently married!" she said. I congratulated her and asked when the wedding was in relation to the onset of her eye problem. She explained that the problem came up before the wedding. However, she had been going through a divorce at the time, which had been contentious, with its finality in question right up to the date of her recent wedding. I nodded, and before I could ask anything further, she reported that she had been under additional pressure: She had lost her job, her son had serious dental problems that she couldn't afford to have treated, and her mother had been hospitalized for a heart problem. She said she was terribly concerned and couldn't see their futures clearly. What became apparent was that her medical signs and symptoms mirrored the circumstances of her life and her story. Her physical manifestations were in some way related to her biographic, mental, and emotional distress. While we can't make solid cause and effect determinations about her situation, it is hard to deny that the stress in one's life plays a significant role in situations such as hers.

This case history illustrates how the immune system is challenged by life events, and how these events and our response to them create our stories of health and healing. For example, a common time for students to get sick is during final exams, and one of the most frequent times for a heart attack is when people return to work on Monday morning. On the other hand, psychosocial support can contribute to survival in cancer patients, married men live longer than unmarried men, and those who believe they will live a long time often do. These phenomena reveal how the story you live and the stories you tell yourself contribute to your health or lack of it.

HEALING CONNECTIONS

To elucidate how stories relate to a person's healing path, and how they can inspire healing in others, consider this: Every person's story is about connection, not only to family ancestry but to the collective as well. For example, my story, and my Jewish roots, link me directly to an ancient spiritual tradition. My experience with oppression and slavery is not merely a biblical tale but literally genetic. My understanding of genocide and annihilation goes beyond this nation's shared history of pioneers immigrating to America for a new life and impacting the lives of indigenous peoples in the process. The reality of attempted genocide lives in my story through my unknown relatives who were stripped of all they had and displaced or killed during the Holocaust during World War II. By extension, descendants of African-American slaves, native peoples who have seen their traditions destroyed and their lands confiscated and degraded, and immigrants who are exploited and disrespected because of their differentness also point to stories and traditions that are either health creating or health negating in their implications and impacts.

Beyond fostering a sense of service or fairness or sympathy, these connections can stimulate compassion for others and oneself. Our connections can be traced back past the judgments, prejudices, and fears that fuel resistance to what we don't understand or accept.

Tracing your roots, telling your story, and hearing the stories of others are actions that lead to healing for both teller and listener. This is about showing up and being present to the story of your life. This is deep medicine.

THE CRACKED POT

The bridge linking the relevance of your personal story to your healing is something you must create for yourself. Your story need not be epic or classic. And melodrama, soap operas, travelogues, and lab reports aren't likely to be the stories that facilitate true healing. That task demands stories that are honest, simple, and authentically your own, and that are heard in an openhearted, fully present way. The significance of the healing nature of our stories can be understood in the following tale, which reveals that what we see in ourselves as defects, flaws, or difficulties can often bear unexpected fruit. Disappointment and perceived shortcomings can lead us onto productive new paths or stimulate growth in new directions, as illustrated by this wonderful fable:

> *A water bearer in India had two large pots, one hanging on each end of a pole that he carried across his shoulders. One of the pots was perfect and always delivered a full portion of water at the end of the long walk from the stream to the master's house, while the other was cracked and arrived only half full. For two years this went on daily, with the bearer delivering only one and a half pots of water to his master's house.*
>
> *Of course, the perfect pot was proud of its accomplishments and how perfectly it fulfilled its purpose. The poor cracked pot, on the other hand, was ashamed of its imperfection and miserable that*

it was able to accomplish only half of what it had been made to do.

After two years of what it perceived to be a bitter failure, it spoke to the water bearer one day by the stream. "I am ashamed of myself," it said, "and I want to apologize to you."

"Why?" asked the bearer. "What are you ashamed of?"

"For these past two years, I have only been able to deliver half of my load because this crack in my side causes water to leak out all the way back to your master's house. Because of my flaws, you don't get the full value from your efforts," the pot said.

The water bearer listened to the old cracked pot, and then compassionately said, "As we return to the master's house, I would like you to notice the beautiful flowers along the path." Indeed, as they went up the hill, the old cracked pot took notice of the sun warming the beautiful wildflowers on the side of the path, and this cheered it some. But at the end of the trail, it still felt bad because it had leaked out half its load, and so once again, it apologized to the water bearer for its failure.

The bearer said to the pot, "Did you notice that there were flowers only on your side of the path, not on the other pot's side? That's because I have always known about your flaw, and I took advantage of it. I planted flower seeds on your side of the path, and every day while we walked back from the stream, you have watered them. For two years I have been able to pick these beautiful flowers to decorate my master's table. Without you being just the way you are, he would not have this beauty to grace his house."

The moral of this story is that each of us has our unique flaws, and that by acknowledging and working with them, rather than regretting them, we can create much beauty in life.

FROM INDIVIDUAL TO UNIVERSAL

Your personal ecology and your social environment both determine the effect of any given stimulus on your health. In *Why People Don't Heal and How They Can* (1997), medical intuitive and best-selling author Carolyn Myss, Ph.D., explains that biology and biography are inseparable. In other words, your reaction to any particular stimulus is dictated not only by your physiological bodily responses, but also by your individual story.

Whether you are aware of it or not, your story informs the big picture as your personal microcosm contributes to the macrocosm—socially, globally, and beyond. Your story is a strand in the unfolding evolution of human consciousness, and sharing stories leads to healing as you discover commonalities and your place in the web of life that sustains us all, no matter what our stage of life or health.

You face different issues and demands during each stage of your life. Physical, mental, emotional, and spiritual issues during each phase of development are different for each individual and vary according to underlying needs affected by circumstances, from genetic to environmental.

The work of two lifelong students of philosopher Rudolf Steiner helps illustrate how phases of life contribute to the creation of your personal story and connect it to the larger picture. In *The Human Life* (1990), George and Gisela O'Neil delineate three main phases: From birth to about twenty years of age, bodily maturity is accomplished. For about the next twenty years, emotional and psychological stability develop. And thereafter, individual and spiritual maturity may follow.

From the perspective of *Deep Medicine*'s theme that everything you think, feel, say, or do is either health creating or health negating, it's clear that successful or appropriate behavior during one stage won't necessarily work at another time, and that inadequate preparation during an early phase may leave you unready for a later one. Each developmental stage builds on the previous one, and all steps are important in order for you to evolve in healthy ways. Where you are underdeveloped or overdeveloped, where you are out of balance, is likely to be reflected in your state of well-being, and in your story. For example, are you physically exhausted, emotionally overwrought, consumed by your work, or living too much in your head? Do you carry what has happened to you during your life as a victim, or do you see yourself as a student, always learning even through painful experiences? Beliefs can be limiting or expanding. Feeling as though you're a victim is a belief that can limit your growth and the potential for healing. Eliminating this and other limiting beliefs may be an important resources for your personal healing project. This is where knowing your story becomes a healing path.

Individual responses fail to neatly fit into predicted patterns, despite our best efforts to create generalizations about what makes us healthy or ill or how any particularly defined group or type will respond to everything from medications and specific foods to environmental factors and prayer. In the final analysis, we are predictable only to a point, and the future is beyond forecasting. We each have our own special wisdom and gifts—our own medicine—to bring to our own healing, to share, and sometimes to endure.

Sources for the deep well-being you seek can be found within your biology and chronology, as well as in your progress on your spiritual path. This seeking requires reenvisioning and revitalizing your inner state of being, not just your outer state of doing!

STORY AS TRANSFORMATION

Each of us has struggles, opinions, points of view, beliefs, and blind spots. Everyone demonstrates repeated behavior patterns, habits, and conditioned responses. Everyone lives with stories: stories we are told and stories we tell. These stories—how we describe ourselves to others, and how we interpret the stories of others—can be constructive or destructive, health creating or health negating. Indeed, as we noted with the metaphors of chapter 3, how you describe a situation, in and of itself, contributes to defining the situation and how you respond to it.

In this light, our stories often need to change, and fortunately they can. For example, you have the power to change your story from a grievance in which you are the victim to a tale of transformation in which you are the shape-shifter or agent of change. As dysfunctional stories shift, you will change, and heal, your reality.

In the form of change talk and resistance talk, storytelling can either strengthen and inspire you and move you to action, or undermine and stifle you and obstruct your growth. You must always be vigilant about the stories you're telling others and the stories you're telling yourself. Remember, your self-talk can build you up or tear you down, so choose to focus on stories that you want to happen. Create constructive possibilities with your self-talk, not tales that feed your fears and doubts or that foster resentment and conflict.

As your stories change, your outlook and your responses to yourself and to others will be transformed.

A Personal Reflection

Some stories in my life have required rewriting, or at least reinterpretation, as times, circumstances, and even people have changed. When the Institute for Health and Healing and its precursor programs were evolving at the California Pacific Medical Center in San Francisco, I often saw myself as a rebel or freedom fighter: a marginalized radical advancing principles and practices that the entrenched medical hierarchy didn't want to hear or see. I had obstacles to circumnavigate, walls to climb, and barriers to break down. It felt like a struggle, a battle. I often spoke of the resistance I was encountering, how people didn't get it, and how little support I was getting.

This was a story I really believed. Well, I believed it as long as I could. But eventually the facts forced me to change my belief. The institute actually received its initial start-up grant from the medical center. The center's philanthropic foundation added us to its organization chart so we had a home, and it raised thousands of dollars for us. Space, overhead support, and administrative salaries were provided by the medical center. Not long after I stopped doing surgery so I could become the full-time medical director of the institute, I was invited onto the medical center's senior management team.

Didn't it seem about time to change my story? Could I still pretend to be a rebel with a cause when anyone objectively looking at what was going on would appropriately conclude that the institute had become a vital, valued part of the medical center's vision and mission? What part of me was unable to trust the creative unfolding that was occurring? What kind of arrogance did this mistrust reveal in me? Of course I was passionate about my dream of holistic medicine becoming a part of contemporary medical practice at major, established medical centers. Even so, I could hardly expect to control every twist and turn of this emerging.

A host of questions and issues called for self-reflection. What was my capacity to trust? My need to control? My self-worth, sufficiency, fear of failure, and level of commitment to my dream all begged for attention. This level of self-searching and self-diagnosis, with or without expert guidance, is necessary for each of us in order to reach a deep level of health and healing. Without this deep and often painful inner work, no self-improvement program will succeed in a sustainable way. This kind of search and discovery mission—examining your beliefs and the stories you tell yourself—is self-empowering and will help you overcome those aspects of your experience that have misinformed you, just as it did for me.

Self-inquiry will help you find the presence of mind and authenticity to recognize and follow your healing path—which isn't an easy task, given the brainwashing delivered daily by agents of consumerism, political spinmeisters, and so-called opinion makers. There is great freedom and hope available in viewing yourself clearly and setting expectations that aren't confined by self-limiting stories or cultural dictates.

A Story to Change

Making the transition to a new story is a powerful way of transforming your life. It need not be major surgery, however; sometimes a subtle or gentle realignment is all that's required.

Several years ago, my wife, Susy, and I had the good fortune to visit Ireland on retreat with the late Celtic poet, theologian, and philosopher John O'Donohue. One day as we hiked the evocative landscape near John's boyhood home, I was struggling with an old story that I considered to be of cultural origin. It concerned the belief I held that if things were going well, they were bound to turn bad. I was moved to ask John about this, appreciating that the Irish people had experienced much hardship and misery in their history. I was wondering if he harbored a similar belief.

He acknowledged the pervasiveness of this story, which is based in fear and can lead to worry and concern even in joyful times because of an ingrained belief that things will inevitably take a turn for the worse. John suggested a revision to this story. His version was that at times when things are going so wonderfully well, it may be too good to be true. However, it is what it is. In this version it is enough to be joyful, uplifted, and grateful for the goodness, not worrying about the transient nature of our well-being and good fortune. Although beliefs and ideas aren't always easy to change, sometimes even a subtle change in perspective—or even just the willingness to make a change—can make a big difference in our well-being. In this case, adjusting my story changed my attitude about impermanence and relieved some of my anxiety about things over which I had no control anyway.

In his book *Journey of Awakening* (1990), Ram Dass tells a story about a king who sequestered his wisest advisors, challenging them to come up with the secret of what can make us happy when we are sad and sad when we are happy. The advisors, stimulated by the threat of execution if they couldn't solve the riddle, came up with four words that solved the dilemma: "This too shall pass." This remains wise counsel even today, as we face the uncertainty of tomorrow.

It isn't only small changes in attitudes, perspectives, stories, and beliefs that work this magic and help create health; making small changes in a well-traveled route or your daily schedule also can lead to a greater flexibility in habits of thinking and action that, over time, will create the healing transformation you seek. It's all about becoming aware of your ways of doing and of being. Knowing yourself and your story is part of what will lead you to the right place at the right time. It will also help you recognize when to quit and when you need to persist, even if the going is tough.

Shake It Off and Step Up

Listen to stories, fables, and myths with care, especially those you tell yourself over and over as reasons why you can't, won't, don't, shouldn't, or should. As you examine your stories, take inspiration from this parable about a farmer and his old mule.

One unfortunate day, the old mule fell into a deep, dry well. The farmer heard the mule's piteous braying and noted an unusual amount of distress in the tenor of his cries. Upon discovering his mule's sad plight, the farmer became quite upset. Tears came to his eyes and his heart ached. He loved all his animals, especially that old mule.

After carefully assessing the situation, the farmer realized the well was a safety hazard. He became angry with himself for not closing off the well and preventing such an accident. But sadly, he could think of no way to extricate his beloved mule from the depths of the well.

The farmer called his neighbors together and told them what had happened. He then enlisted them to help haul dirt to fill up the well and, at the same time, put his old mule out of his misery.

Initially, the old mule became more hysterical as the dirt was thrown upon his back. But as the farmer and his neighbors continued shoveling, inspiration struck and the mule realized he could shake off the dirt and take a step up. This he did, blow after blow, repeating, "Shake it off, and step up. Shake it off, and step up. Shake it off, and step up..."

Time after time after time he repeated this mantra to encourage himself, and no matter how painful the blows from the dirt, or how distressing the situation seemed, the old mule fought panic and kept right on shaking the dirt off and stepping up, climbing higher and higher in the process.

It wasn't long before the old mule, battered and exhausted, stepped triumphantly out of the well.

As Winston Churchill reportedly said, when you're going through hell, keep on going.

GOING BEYOND THE PERSONAL

For each of us, our individual story begins with an inherited genetic map and the circumstances we are born into. We all have tales of the trials, tribulations, and treasures of our upbringing and family of origin. Some of what you are and will be has been already cast and is beyond your influence. Nonetheless, a good bit of your story can be influenced. How you respond to what happens to you or has happened to you is in large part under your jurisdiction. How you see and engage your present set of circumstances and how you prepare for and dream the future are also within your purview.

My power to heal and effect change lies in my good fortune of privilege and position, and in my passion to express and share my gifts and talents in a way that goes beyond myself and my immediate family. Exploring my story is part of my healing journey and strengthens my capacity to contribute to the healing of others. Through story I have entered into the collective conversation of how together we can be forces of healing (wholeness) rather than of separation or disease. A similar healing story is available to you if you seek it, though its manifestation will, of course, reflect your unique character and circumstances.

The key is that to engage this healing story, you need to show up at the party, flaws and all. Being fully present *is* a present; it's a gift you give yourself, and a gift you offer to every encounter, situation, and relationship in which you are involved.

No healer, no matter how talented, knowledgeable, or intuitive, can ever know you as well as you know yourself. Through self-knowledge, you will develop great power to effect your own healing. While you can, and often should, seek help from others (doctors, friends, teachers, clergy, and other healers), you must use your self-knowledge to understand which lifestyle patterns are health enhancing for you and which are health negating. Then you must make choices. Decide what to do and what not to do, when to push forward and when to hold back. The tools for change in chapter 3 and the pillars and practices in chapter 4—and the tools and practices you develop on your own—are the source of your healing powers. They will nourish your well-being and support your outer actions as you travel your own unique path to creating health.

EXERCISE FOR CHAPTER 5: WHAT'S YOUR STORY, AND ARE YOU STICKING TO IT?

Exercise 1: Hearing and Changing Your Stories

What stories do you tell yourself that keep you from what you desire? That you don't have time for healthful practices, that you can't afford them, or that you'll start down your healing path soon—next week, next month, next year? Listen to these recurring excuses, rationalizations, explanations, and stories. Listen carefully to your language and the terms you choose to describe yourself and others. Then track their source and be prepared to change the story!

Exercise 2: What Drains You? What Fills You?

Making health-enhancing decisions requires personal knowledge of what fills you and what depletes you. In order to set your priorities and pursue them with intention and honesty, ask yourself the following questions:

🌱 Who am I? What am I seeking?

🌱 What is motivating me to seek?

🌱 Am I my physical body, my feelings and sensations, my personality, my inner observer, my soul?

- Do I really stop at the limits of my skin?

- How far does my mind or consciousness reach?

- What of my ancestral roots? What is the background of my name?

- Who were my parents?

- What were their hopes?

- What were their fears?

- What were their dreams?

- What were their thoughts and feelings about work and play? Health and illness? Conflict and anger? How did they deal with these issues?

- What are my thoughts about these issues, and how do I deal with them?

Exercise 3: What Are You Tired Of?

Have you ever said or thought, "That makes me sick!" or "I am so tired of..."? Can you identify certain circumstances that literally make you sick? Can you identify behavior patterns that repeatedly lead you to those circumstances? Is there anything you could do to avoid those circumstances?

Exercise 4: Building Your Story

Here are some questions and suggestions to reflect upon in building your own story of health and well-being:

- How does your story fit with the big picture and with your legacy?

- Honor your past, and consider creating a family tree. What can you learn about yourself and your story from your past history?

- Why are you presently living where you are living? Why are you working where you do? Does probing your geography and placement open any doors for you?

- Envision your future—a future of health and well-being, a future in which anything is possible for you. If you can dream it, you can manifest it if you act on it.

- Invite others to tell you their story, and listen with your heart as well as your ears.

Exercise 5: The Theme of Your Life Story

Your personal story has such a profound capacity to create or negate healing that it's worthwhile to examine it from many perspectives. Here are some additional questions to guide you in reflecting on your circumstances and your life story:

☙ Is there a message or a theme?

☙ Is there an underlying truth?

☙ Is there a payoff? What's in it for you?

☙ Are your chronic symptoms (backache, headache, stomach pain, whatever) related to the load you're presently carrying, something that may be a pain in the back or a pain in the neck, or that hits you in your gut?

☙ Has a health condition or illness taught you something about yourself that you were denying, avoiding, or unable to see, and thus led you to change your life?

☙ Do your symptoms help you get attention or sympathy, or allow you to escape from difficult or unsatisfactory situations?

☙ Can illness be more than an obstacle or a challenge?

☙ Can illness be a wake-up call, an activator, or an opening?

CHAPTER 6

Making the Connection from Personal Health to Planetary Healing

As is the human body, so is the cosmic body.
As is the human mind, so is the cosmic mind.
As is the microcosm, so is the macrocosm.
As is the atom, so is the universe.

—The Upanishads

See the world as yourself.
Have faith in the way things are.
Love the world as yourself;
Then you can care for all things.

—Lao Tzu

Your personal health-creating practices profoundly influence the unfolding of your life story. What also needs to be brought to awareness is the powerful ripple effect that your story has beyond your own life. You must see your story in the context of your relationship to all around you, including Planet Earth. Your story individualizes the big picture and makes the global personal. Rediscovering and reclaiming your intimate connection to Mother Earth is practicing deep medicine, and a critical part of the wholeness and balance that define true well-being.

Further evolution of human consciousness, both individually and collectively, is necessary if we are to truly and fully move beyond the limitations of tribalism and personal prejudices. Each of us can forward that evolution through personal growth and healing. As we explored in chapter 5, tracing our roots, telling our stories, hearing the stories of others, and understanding ourselves in relationship to everything around us will help us define the similarities, commonalities, and connections that lead to healing change at all levels, from the personal to the global.

Scientific data and cultural wisdom inform us that we have an intimate relationship with the Earth such that the health of the individual person is inseparable from that of the planet. In the fast-paced lifestyle of the twenty-first century, we have lost sight of this reality. However, without an awareness of the deep connection between individual health and well-being and that of our environment and planet, we cannot hope to be truly well, nor can we anticipate that our Earth will be healthy. We will also be unable to develop the loving relationships that anchor a full and healthy life.

PLANETARY HEALTH

In our modern world, we are faced with a daily onslaught of examples of planetary degradation that directly impact our health: air pollution, ozone depletion, global warming, water contamination and shortages, topsoil erosion, rain forest destruction, interspecies infections, human overpopulation, and the threat of nuclear disaster. This tabulation, though incomplete, reads like the table of contents of a medical book describing the various states of disease of the planetary body. Not surprisingly, this ever-expanding list of environmental ills is reflected in the catalog of congenital deformities, infections and infestations, degenerative diseases, fluid and electrolyte imbalances, nutritional deficiencies, respiratory maladies, psychological illnesses, and cancers that plague our bodies in lockstep with the destruction of our environment.

Our intimate relationship with the Earth is emphasized not only by our shared maladies, but also by significant physiological commonalities. The proportion of water in our bodies is about the same as that on the Earth's surface. The concentration of salt in our blood is similar to that in the oceans. The proportion of oxygen in the atmosphere allows aerobic reactions to occur without uncontrolled combustion. The universe is expanding fast enough that the force of gravity doesn't pull everything back together, but slowly enough that we don't fly off into the vastness of space.

These and other microscopic and macroscopic relationships between our species and our natural world remind us of our planetary heritage. We are of the planet, not just on it. From this vantage point, we can see the Earth as a whole—like the now familiar blue-green image from space—and appreciate our planet as the living organism that it is.

The challenge of maintaining our planet's delicate balance of life-sustaining systems is truly the health care issue of our time. Our precious planet provides the only potable water, fertile topsoil, and oxygen-containing atmosphere within over a trillion miles. There isn't a backup planet!

My early and idealistic desire to create the first "Department of Planetary Medicine" at a major medical center contributed to the beginnings of what is now the Institute for Health and Healing in San Francisco. During my scientific and medical training, I had become aware of the exquisite biological, chemical, mathematical, and physics-based relationships that allow for the miracle of life on this planet. The elegance, intelligence, and beauty of the interplay and the integrated whole moved me deeply—and continues to do so.

As a physician, father, and grandfather, I am compelled to foster and promote an appreciation of the value and power of these relationships. Understanding and honoring these delicate environmental balances makes each of us physicians to the Earth. More than other species, humans have the capacity to safeguard the balance and restore equilibrium; we are vital elements in the equation.

Appreciating the mystery, magic, and complexity of these delicate and life-supporting relationships also makes us priests and priestesses of the Earth. In their book *The Universe Story* (1992), cosmologist Brian Swimme and Father Thomas Berry suggest that humans are literally the consciousness or awareness of the planet. Because we are an integral part of the planet, when we care about what is happening to the Earth, the Earth is caring for itself. The next time some troublesome skeptic asks you if the Earth really cares about _____ (fill in the blank with, for example, melting of the polar icecaps, greenhouse gases, destroying the rain forests, extirpating species), you can legitimately answer, "Yes!" If we care, the Earth cares.

A COSMIC VIEW OF WHERE WE ARE

Looking at the planet as an integrated whole, and at humans as a part of that whole, usually requires a shift in perspective. Swimme has said that if we really knew where we were, we would know how to behave. American Jewish writer and newspaper publisher Harry Golden, in *Only in America*, writes about how an astronomer's view of the cosmos helps put things in perspective (1958, p. 21):

> *I have a rule against registering complaints in a restaurant, because I know that there are at least four billion suns in the Milky Way—which is only one galaxy. Many of these suns are thousands of times larger than our own, and vast millions of them have whole planetary systems... Our own sun and its planets, which include this Earth, are on the edge of...space...so unbelievably vast that if we reduced the suns and the planets in correct mathematical proportions with relation to the distances between them, each sun*

would be a speck of dust, two, three, and four thousand miles away from its nearest neighbor. And mind you, this is only the Milky Way—our own small corner—our own galaxy. How many galaxies are there? Billions... When you think of all this, it's silly to worry about whether the waitress brought you string beans instead of limas.

Each of us is but a small part of a much larger picture. You should never forget that reality, especially during times when your personal issues loom particularly large. In her book *Happiness is an Inside Job* (2007), popular storyteller and Buddhist teacher Sylvia Boorstein likens the interplay of each human life with the bigger picture to the picture-in-picture option on a television, which allows simultaneous viewing of multiple shows on one screen. Your individual story is playing in a small box on the screen, against the backdrop of the story of the planet.

The Need for Broader Perspective

The magnitude and pace of human development, particularly in the realm of science and technology, must also be seen in their moral, ethical, and compassionate dimensions. From space travel to medical breakthroughs to digital communications, our human accomplishments are significant. But amidst these grandiose accomplishments, a significant proportion of the human population is chronically malnourished, there is an increasing disparity between haves and have-nots, violent crimes occur at unprecedented levels, and more attention and resources are devoted to prisons than to public schools. We face increasing individual and planetary illness because of pressures from issues such as population growth, toxic wastes, economic disparity, and climate change.

These global concerns are relevant personal health issues for each of us. Our healing, individually and collectively, depends on addressing the growing disparity between our rapidly expanding knowledge base and technologies and our moral and ethical development. This disparity can be health negating on both personal and planetary levels.

Remember, everything is either health creating or health negating, and everything is connected. Using the example of depending on oil as our primary energy source, it becomes apparent that the health implications extend beyond the cost in terms of direct environmental degradation from air pollution, oil spills, and the like. Global climate change, geopolitical instability, economic woes, and the short-sighted failure to research and develop alternative, renewable energy sources also pose significant threats to our health, well-being, and quality of life, and to the health of our planet.

Consider the wisdom of Chief Seattle, a nineteenth-century leader of the Suquamish tribe in what is now Washington State: "This we know: the Earth does not belong to man; man belongs to the Earth… All things are connected, like the blood which unites one family… Whatever befalls the Earth befalls the sons of the Earth. Man did not weave the web of life; he is merely a strand in it. Whatever he does to the web, he does to himself" (Marshall 1996, p. 141).

Long before the advent of contemporary scientific thinking, many indigenous peoples lived in harmony with their environment. Our modern way of life and rapidly increasing numbers have robbed us of the kind of relationships our forebears had with their environment and the planet. How many of us are intimately familiar with the terrain where we live, our local watershed, and the local flora and fauna? Who among us has a concept of the food chain in our area? How different would your life be if you were as fully in tune with your surroundings as indigenous peoples who live close to the land and sea?

As you consider Chief Seattle's words, also recall the myths from divergent cultures that chronicle honorable, respectful, and compassionate ways of relating to and coexisting with the Earth. The pace and pattern of your life and the status of your health can benefit from this perspective, from learning to honor your connection to the billions of years of creative metamorphosis that have formed this universe, solar system, and planet. I am not suggesting a return to cave and candle, but rather an adjustment in perspective that would allow us to fully see how we're related to the planet, and to value and attend to that relationship in health-creating ways.

Big Rocks

Appreciating our place in the cosmic scheme of things can help us make sound decisions that will foster health and well-being. When we're able to see our planetary impact, we have a greater awareness of what impacts us individually. My friend Sandra Hobson shared the following anecdote with me, about the importance of seeing things in proper perspective:

One day an expert in time management was speaking to a group of business students, and to drive home a point, he used an illustration those students will never forget. As he stood in front of the group of high-powered achievers he said, "Okay, time for a quiz."

He pulled out a one-gallon, wide-mouthed jar and set it on the table in front of him. Then he produced about a dozen fist-sized rocks and carefully placed them, one at a time, in the jar.

When the jar was filled to the top and no more rocks would fit inside, he asked, "Is this jar full?"

When everyone in the class said yes, he said, "Really?" He reached under the table and pulled out a bucket of gravel, then he dumped some gravel in and shook the jar, which allowed some of the gravel to work its way down into the spaces between the big rocks. Then he asked the group once more, "Is this jar full?"

By this time, the class was on to him. "Probably not," one of them answered. "Good!" he replied. He reached under the table and brought out a bucket of sand. He started dumping the sand in the jar, and it flowed into all of the spaces left between the rocks and the gravel. Once more he asked the question, "Is this jar full?" and the class shouted, "No!" Next he brought out a pitcher of water and poured it in until the jar was filled to the brim. Then he looked at the class and asked, "What is the point of this demonstration?"

One eager beaver raised his hand and said, "The point is, no matter how full your schedule is, if you try really hard you can always fit more into it!"

"No," the speaker replied, "that's not the point. The truth this demonstration teaches is that if you don't put the big rocks in first, you'll never get them in at all!"

What are the big rocks in your life? Your loved ones, your health, your education, your dreams, a worthy cause, teaching or mentoring others, doing things you love, taking time for yourself, riding your Harley-Davidson? Remember to put those big rocks in first, or you'll never get them in at all.

If you only focus on the small stuff (the gravel and the sand), you'll fill your life with little things that may or may not be essential, and you'll never have the quality time you need to devote to the big, important things. So take a planetary perspective, then ask yourself this question: "What are the big rocks in my life?" Those are the things you want to put in your jar first.

WHAT TIME IS IT?

Taking the planetary perspective, in both time and space, gives us reason to make the most of our conscious moments in all the domains of our lives. Every generation of humans considers their time to be an age of challenge, filled with amazing developments, and this seems particularly relevant to our time. What has happened in the last one hundred years makes the previous one thousand or twenty thousand years look like dormancy. One hundred years ago, transportation, communication, and ecological disaster meant riding your horse into town and stopping at the general store to talk about the creek overflowing its banks. Today, we telecommunicate with all corners of the globe, access the archives of human knowledge, and destroy far reaches of the planet in the blink of an eye. Our human pace has become mind-boggling and often overwhelming.

We can take comfort from a planetary perspective, in which time is measured in epochs and eons, and from a spiritual perspective that time is eternal. To paraphrase an ancient Hindu text, the Bhagavad Gita (Easwaran 2000), having been (existing in some form now), you always were, and always will be. And although from the vantage point of our daily lives time is measured in minutes, hours, days, and years, from a scientific perspective time is relative. However we conceive of time, our individual existence is transient. All aspects of creation demonstrate a dynamic impermanence, moving through birth, growth, maturation, decline, death, and decay. While all of these stages are sure to occur, when and how is an individual mystery that lends an element of uncertainty to our lives.

This impermanence is one of the strong arguments for aware, awake, mindful living in the present moment. We never really know which moment will be our last, nor when loss, tragedy, or good fortune will appear or disappear. This awareness of impermanence is also an underpinning of one of *Deep Medicine*'s themes: the importance and the challenge of change. When we apply this awareness to a more global context and see everything as transitory and impermanent, we can truly shift perspective in a way that just might lead us to be more merciful, generous, and composed.

Love Is the Answer

We simultaneously and repeatedly enter and exit, give and receive, hold onto and let go, seek the new and discard the used, gain and lose, grow and decay, get injured and heal, hurt and forgive. It is the nature of our existence to grow and change over time. Even as we experience the joy of watching our children grow, they are leaving us. Living fully now is the best insurance against the tragedy of an unlived or unfulfilled life.

Finding your place in the scheme of things and living in a way that appropriately frames your relationship to the planet is part of practicing deep medicine. Feeling the intimate connection that you share with this planet and all of its communities is part of harnessing the source of your healing power. It is said that the practice of relationship is all any of us needs for our spiritual journey. And indeed, appreciating and living the differences between falling in love (egoism, romance, and fantasy), being in love (commitment, loyalty, and shared goals), and staying in love (growth, change, and partnership) provides fertile ground for character development, awareness, and expanding consciousness, as does recognizing the differences between a mother's love for her child, love between partners, love for one's vocation or avocation, and love for a pet, fine music, or surfing.

To love requires curiosity and understanding, communication and creativity, honor and respect. These characteristics define not only your relationship with your self, your family and friends, your collectives, and the sacred, but also your relationship with the planet—your Mother Earth—as well. Nothing short of a loving relationship will allow us a healing partnership with our planet, and with ourselves.

EXERCISES FOR CHAPTER 6: PERSONAL HEALTH AND PLANETARY HEALING

Exercise 1: Your Relationship with Earth

Reflect on your own personal relationship with the planet. (Hint: It's not called Mother Earth for nothing.) Here are a few specific questions to guide your contemplation:

- Where did your lunch come from? (And I don't mean Dave's Deli.) Where will it go?

- When you say, "Throw it away," where is away?

- Can the effects of your daily habits be separate from the planet, or do you see yourself and your actions and lifestyle choices as part of the food chain?

Exercise 2: The Environmental Web

Consider the role of mankind in these large-scale disasters:

- Drought and famine in Africa

- Global warming

- Respiratory disease in Los Angeles

- Chernobyl in the former USSR

Consider the health implications of these alternative approaches:

- Mass transit

- Recycling

- Organic farming

- Renewable energy

Exercise 3: Humanity's Place in the Web

Revisit the words from Chief Seattle that appeared in this chapter, about the web of life and humanity's place within that web. Was (is) he correct? In what small ways might you become more aware on a daily basis of your interconnectedness with the Earth and, by extension, humanity's interconnectedness with the Earth?

Exercise 4: What Time Is It?

Where are you and what time is it for you? Is it the right place and the right time? If not, what do you need to do to make it so?

Exercise 5: The Evolution of Being

Consider the following relational sequences in the context of the evolutionary history of the planet:

Subatomic particles —> molecules —> cells —> tissues —>
organs —> systems —> organisms

Elements —> matter —> life —> mind —> consciousness

Individual —> family —> tribe —> city —> state —> nation —>
humankind

What do these sequences mean to you? Is there a relationship or evolutionary arc from the microcosm to the macrocosm? Where do you fit in? Do you fit into more than one place?

Consider the statement "Personal well-being leads to the public health, which leads to planetary healing." Does it make sense to you? And how is this statement related to the sequences above?

CHAPTER 7

Bridging Inner and Outer Worlds and Becoming Whole

What lies behind us and what lies before us are small matters compared to what lies within us.

—Ralph Waldo Emerson

What we plant in the soil of contemplation, we shall reap in the harvest of action.

—Meister Eckhart

When I was in a sophomore in high school, I wrote a paper on Darwin's theory of evolution and the book of Genesis. As might be expected, it was a sophomoric paper, but it was also an early attempt to bring together opposites—in this case divergent explanations of the creation of life from scientific and sacred perspectives. Becoming whole, balanced, or healthy often requires seeing the complementarity in knowledge and practices that may hail from different or even seemingly opposite sources, cultures, systems, and perspectives. For example, surgery, chemotherapy, acupuncture, massage, guided imagery, and prayer may all be used—and useful—in the treatment of a serious illness. That is holistic medicine—medicine that treats the whole person. This movement toward wholeness is the true work of health and healing.

Forwarding this work is deep medicine's ultimate purpose.

Many years ago, the tensions between creationists and evolutionists stimulated me to come to terms with competing explanations of the existence of the universe and of humanity. By engaging this dissonance and the struggle to merge two opposing positions, I brought something very difficult to understand into a construct that made sense to me and found a relationship with the mystery of creation that continues to serve me. This was a compromise around a synthesis that acknowledged the difficulty—actually the discomfort or pain—associated with trying to explain the unexplainable.

A significant part of healing involves reducing pain and suffering. And part of this healing process means negotiating the creative tension of paradox. My own early step in dealing with paradox began a lifelong willingness to hold seeming opposites that has been healing. The exercise of writing that high school paper reduced the "suffering" I felt because of being unable to fully explain reality and helped me accept paradox and mystery.

My work as a surgeon has placed me at the interface of science and spirit. Being able to hold paradox has affected how I practice medicine and how I view and honor the potential for positive change inherent in every health crisis or challenge. On the one hand, surgery is a precise anatomical and technological activity demanding the best science can offer. On the other hand, it is a priestly activity supported by ritual, including hand washing and wearing "ceremonial" operating room gowns. Trusting patients, anesthetized upon the operating table, give themselves over to the surgical team. The cold stainless steel blade pierces the flesh, allowing entry to the hallowed bodily core. Probing exploration, excision of diseased tissue, and repair of injury occur amid the pulsing warmth of bodily organs and fluids. The surgeon is not only a technician of the flesh, but also an instrument of healing and of care. The healing impact of the surgeon's kind words, eye contact, smile, and gentle touch has power, just as the knife and the laser do.

Bringing together science and the sacred means bringing together the outer, rational, physical world and the inner, subjective, spiritual world. Your path to health and healing mandates opening yourself to the unknown. Appreciating the uncertainty and transient nature of your existence in its outer, physical, temporal form and the enduring, external nature of existence in its inner, spiritual, and sacred aspects contributes to realizing the source of your healing power. Integrating your outer and inner worlds is necessary to becoming whole. Therefore, this bridging is another essential ingredient in the practice of deep medicine, in motivating you to use the tools of change and the pillars and practices of well-being, all with the goal of harnessing the source of your healing power.

Contemporary medicine may be the bridge, the interface, between the best of applied science and the deepest questions about the meaning of our existence. For here we bring together our inner, sacred, soulful parts with our physical, material, and rational parts and go beyond our physical bodies to enhance the potential for health and healing. Here the elements of our spirituality are brought into play. As our physical, bodily reality is challenged by illness and infirmity, our faith, belief systems, and capacity to trust are also tested. Values are called into high relief as the worth of our material possessions pales in comparison to the gift of health. It is vital for contemporary medicine to bridge science and spirit; however, the ultimate key to healing is for each of us to bridge our outer and inner worlds.

Your personal balance or wholeness (health) and the changes you must make to restore that balance (healing) require ways of knowing and the wisdom and power residing in both the outer and inner worlds.

THE POWER OF PARADOX: OPPOSITES ATTRACT

A paradox is a seemingly self-contradictory statement. Generally, paradox relates to a truth, the opposite of which is also true. Paradox is often represented by extremes, dualities, or opposites that coexist and, in fact, turn out to be connected: dark/light, up/down, left/right, inner/outer, logical/emotional, pain/pleasure, rich/poor, order/chaos, health/illness, right/wrong, difficult/easy, good/evil, moral/immoral. Human cultures have many symbols and philosophical constructs that represent the dilemma posed by duality and paradox and the unseen ways they are connected: the yin and the yang, the double-edged sword, the concepts of subjective and objective, the so-called divide between fact and faith, and so on. A French proverb speaks to how deeply paradox is intertwined with our existence, noting that we often meet our destiny on the road we take to avoid it.

Science may act as though it does not need mysticism, and mysticism may seem as though it does not need science, but humanity needs both. Science and spirit are bridged by unseen connections that exist at the liminal edge between what is known and what is unknown. Science is a powerful and flexible instrument in the search for health and truth. Knowledge and skills broaden as new information becomes available through careful and rigorous experimental methods and repeatable observations. When scientists become rigid and inflexible, however, their work is no longer science; it becomes dogma or edict. True science is curious and flexible, encouraging growth and change, and seeing our present limits as temporary boundaries casting what lies beyond as a mystery.

In Western medicine, analytical methods and diagnosis are dominated by outer structure and attention to form. By contrast, in traditional Chinese medicine, the whole is made up of yin and yang, poles that paradoxically oppose and complement each other. Outer manifestations are yang, an external and explicit reality always accompanied by yin, the inner and implicit dimension. Yin characteristics reflect process and the receptive, intuitive, and mysterious sides of things. Yin and yang inform everything, including communication:

Yang talks and yin listens. Relating the two is at the heart of relationship, and seeing the relationships between yin and yang, as well as outer and inner aspects of ourselves, is essential to seeing wholeness.

Similarly, our lives are not limited to the external or yang elements or confines, although we often live as if they were. As we evolve as humans and as healers, we are carried to the vast frontiers of our invisible, inner, yin landscape. The complementary models of yin *and* yang, inner *and* outer, mind *and* body don't require us to choose between scientific and sacred worldviews; rather, they invite us to appreciate the juxtaposition of seeming contradictions. Our health-creating and healing work gives each of us the opportunity to merge these seeming paradoxes on a daily basis.

The personal quest for health brings us face-to-face with many paradoxes and dilemmas. There are splits or separations that might not represent accurate interpretations of the world. For example, even the largest realities can be unseen. The sun is still there even when obscured by clouds, as is a mountain enshrouded in fog. Our understanding of seeing must extend beyond the physical—outside the visible spectrum of electromagnetic energy—to include unseen realms, like the inner world of spirit.

This awareness opens new possibilities and allows us to access a broader range of healing modalities, and rightly so. Can we ever know for sure if it was the chemotherapy or the will to live, the antibiotic or the prayer, the laser treatment or the inspiring words that made the difference between recovery and recurrence?

BEYOND THE KNOWN

What lies beyond the range of our largest telescopes? What might be seen if our strongest microscope had even greater powers of magnification? What exists before birth and after death? These questions touch the hows and whys of our existence, where scientific facts blend with spiritual issues of source and meaning. For a society most comfortable with the objective, the impersonal, and technical facts, the subjective aspects of the world reveal limits and vulnerabilities, but also possibilities, even though they may induce anxiety regarding the unknown. We can't do our work only when it's easy. Consider that the precious pearl is a result of irritation and lies hidden within a protective shell. In creating our health and advancing our healing, we must be willing to experience discomfort, and to venture where it is dark and messy and difficult.

One way of appreciating your inner realm is to acknowledge the unconscious power of intuition, a knowing that comes from unseen sources. Have you had the experience of love at first sight? Have you felt the phenomenon of flow, when everything falls into place effortlessly and you feel a sense of timelessness? Have you entered a room, perhaps where a party or a meeting was going on, and immediately had an energetic sense of what was happening or that you did or did not want to be there? If so, you've had a direct personal experience of the power of intuition and the messages it offers. This is the source of your inner healer, the mysterious yet fertile soil from which your inner wisdom arises.

Living a fully engaged life—one of the hallmarks of good health—requires us to coexist with the uncertainty and anxiety of one of the keystone mysteries of our existence. At some point in the course of our health, illness, and healing, we confront the inevitability and fear of death, and the uncertainty surrounding it. In *The Tibetan Book of Living and Dying* (1992), Buddhist teacher and author Sogyal Rinpoche writes that learning to die is how one truly learns how to live. We fear death in part because of our attachment to the concept of the physical body. Our perceived separation from the natural cycles of nature also distances us from the reality of death. Yet all that surrounds us is impermanent and transitory. Like sunsets and rainbows, neither people nor mountains last forever in one particular form.

Many sources offer descriptions of what happens after life ends. Our beliefs and faith often define our view of this question, and for all we know, death may entail a continuation of life in some undivulged form. It is a mystery. It isn't a puzzle; we won't find a missing piece that explains it all. We exist within an unfinished riddle. The question has been posed, but the solution is unlikely to be revealed anytime soon. This mystery encompasses not only death, but also the time before birth.

Health doesn't mean avoiding death or even necessarily postponing it. Health *does* involve coming to terms with death, though Western society tends to deny this. Consider the popularity of cosmetic surgery, with its facelifts, hair transplants, and tummy tucks, or the plethora of "antiaging" skin creams—and at the extreme end of the spectrum, the cosmetological arts of the funeral parlor. Vast industries have been built on attempts to disguise or postpone the reality of death and its precursors in the form of wrinkles, hair loss, and weight gain. Yet hundreds of thousands of people die each day—millions each year. We all show signs of death's impending, although unpredictable, arrival, as age sculpts our bodies. As a culture, we often view death as an end, a terminal event, a tragedy, a failure, or a loss. In other spiritual traditions, however, death is often viewed as merely leaving the physical body and as much a beginning as an ending. It is seen as another threshold in the mysterious journey of which bodily existence is only one part.

Part of the suffering around the fear of death—and the healing that can arise with an acceptance of death—is that its inevitability is coupled with unpredictability about exactly how and when it will occur. True, someone with end-stage cancer may be more likely to die than a teenage gymnast. However, lightning does strike and remarkable remissions are possible. Not knowing which day or hour will be your last raises the stakes. Life asks that you not waste precious time. You are called to cherish each moment, to value the ordinary and the extraordinary, to use your life well. You need to seize the day, be here now, bring your attention to what's really important, and gratefully honor the gift of time inhabiting a body here on Earth.

When you go beyond the physical to recognize the inner spiritual forces that operate within you, you will see and experience love, meaning, and belief as healing forces as powerful as medications, scalpels, and all of the other tools of conventional medicine. From that perspective, you will understand that no single answer can be right for everyone, and that it's up to you to use this book's tools, pillars, and practices in your own way, with your own agenda, and on your own timeline, with one caveat: Always prioritize the things that are most important to you. Your time is limited and your exact timeline unknown.

BUILDING BRIDGES

By coming to terms with paradox and mystery, you bring yourself a step closer to operating from the perspective of connectedness inherent in deep medicine. Seeing the continuum between what initially appear to be opposites is part of seeing the whole within which we exist. Be open to the possibility that you can learn as much from a small child as from a wise elder, and remember that you can benefit from your failures as well as your successes.

Our common connectedness to all around us through joy, sorrow, empathy, sympathy, and shared human experience cannot be denied. The power of subjective experience and the texture and resilience of our spirituality often inform us with greater accuracy than the objective facts often used to make health-related decisions for ourselves and our loved ones. If Grandma is on a respirator in the intensive care unit, many facts and figures will contribute to decisions such as if and when the respirator and other life support are discontinued— data such as the cost of care, laboratory test results, her chances for survival, and insurance coverage. In the end, however, it is likely that more intangible factors, such as her love of life, her wishes, and her family's weighing of her pain and suffering, will be most critical in making decisions about her care.

As you become more comfortable at the meeting place of the scientific and the spiritual, even some of the most basic scientific tenets can be understood as having profound spiritual implications, in addition to their rational ramifications. In truth, science and spiritual study raise similar concerns and remind us that wholeness and health require a both-and approach, not an either-or mind-set. In *The Universe Story* (1992), cosmologist Brian Swimme and Father Thomas Berry wed contemporary scientific understanding and the world's great wisdom traditions in describing fifteen billion years of cosmic existence. They recount the story of the universe as science and myth, blending geological and biological findings with our search for meaning. In examining Einstein's famous formula $E=mc^2$, in which energy equals mass times the speed of light squared, they explore how something we perceive as pure science—physics and mathematics— also represents a powerful spiritual truth: that energy and matter are the same. What else is there on the planet but energy and matter in their various forms? This is scientific corroboration of the interconnectedness of everything on our planet, and that we are in a constant state of interplay with our surroundings. Recognizing that what we perceive as energy (light, sound, electromagnetic force) and what we perceive as matter (animal, vegetable, mineral, gas, solid, liquid) are related and are in a state of constant flow and interchange is a profound lesson. This understanding connects you to the reality that your personal well-being is always directly and fundamentally related to the state of the planet and reminds you that everything has either a health-creating or health-negating impact on you.

The disciplines of physics, chemistry, mathematics, and biology are no stranger to spiritual questions. Gary Zukav in *The Dancing Wu Li Masters* (1989) and Fritjof Capra in *The Tao of Physics* (1984) both explore and support the concept of a relationship between science and the sacred and between the visible and invisible worlds. Science has taught us that the atomic structure and basic particles of which humans are made—protons, neutrons, and electrons—are identical to those found in all organic and inorganic substances. Various chemical elements (including carbon, hydrogen, and oxygen) and compounds (such as water and salt) are ubiquitous in nature. At a molecular level, significant quantities of DNA are shared—even by very different species. Even our understanding of the seemingly fundamental concept of solidity is brought into question by the scientific explanation of our makeup. Although our sensory perception tells us we are solid within our skin, our atomic particles beg to differ. Relative to the size of the particles that are our building blocks, vast distances of space exist between those particles. At the atomic level, our particles are as distant from one another as the planets and stars are in the expanse of space. We are more empty than solid! Nonetheless, when you sit in a chair, it supports your weight, and you cannot walk through a wall in spite of the inherent open space that resides within both the wall and your body.

Like science, spiritual traditions also bring to light the dynamism and impermanence of our human condition: from dust to dust. It is the nature of our existence to be balanced on the cusp of energy and matter, full of emptiness and in constant flow, dancing the cosmic dance with both science and spirit. The breakfast we ate this morning becomes the energy that fuels our bodies, just as an acorn gains energy from sun, soil, and water. The acorn expresses its potential by becoming the tree that yields the log that feeds the fire that warms our bodies that leaves the ash that returns to soil once again to feed the interconnected, interdependent cycle of which we are a part. There is much to nature's cycles that eludes scientific explanation and leaves us with questions that attempt to penetrate the origins of creation and its unfolding. These questions bring the mystics, mathematicians, philosophers, theologians, and physicists together in search of answers at the interface between scientific inquiry and philosophic dialogue. This is where science and the sacred become inseparable partners, in exploring the questions that form the bridge between the explicit, objective, rational, and material and the realm of the nonmaterial, implicit, subjective, and invisible—in bridging our outer and inner worlds.

Simply stated, we need both science and the sacred to be healthy and whole.

BECOMING THE HEALTHY WHOLE

Clearly, we need to go beyond our physical bodies to understand and fully foster our potential for health, healing, and well-being. We need to explore and gauge the inner, invisible world that might not be discovered by the physician's use of direct observation, palpation, and all manner of technological devices—those recesses of your being that are not necessarily accessed by the usual questions asked by your doctor in regard to your symptoms, chief complaint, and personal and family health history. The inner landscape is the territory of questions such as why am I here, what does it mean, and what purposes do I serve?

The inner landscape cannot be entered through intellect and reason alone. It must be felt by direct spiritual experience. Thus it requires a different kind of knowing than the objective and rational—a knowing that comes through contemplative practice, wisdom study, and direct experience. The intellect and descriptions are necessary, but they aren't capable of fully conveying your direct experiences. Scientific thought seeks theories of things, whereas the pursuit of inner wisdom seeks spiritual discovery, transformation, and realization. The path that leads to the innermost self can be obscured by overthinking, and direct experiences can actually be missed. Therefore, simple contemplative practices that aren't based on objective thought or that actually suspend thinking, such as the deep minute, are necessary, not optional, on the journey to health and healing.

It is somewhere in the coming together of seeming opposites that creativity and abundance live and prosper. The dualities that seem to exist on our planet are quite interesting, curious, and instructive. It is noteworthy how necessary it is for male and female parts (opposites?) to come together for biological reproduction in most species. Is this the ultimate duality? Doesn't it have a paradoxical quality about it? To sustain the species we must bring opposites together. To explain our existence we must make sense of opposites, extremes, and polarities. For example, healers need illness to express their gift of healing, and peacemakers need conflict to bring forward their peacemaking medicine. As we come to recognize the continuum underlying polarities, dualities, opposites, and paradox, we create the crossroads and thresholds where healing occurs. On the bridge between opposite shores we find connection, compromise, creative tension, balance, wholeness, and health in their truest incarnations.

We cherish, seek, and value the heroic, but isn't the humdrum just as important? Inadequate physical activity isn't good for our well-being, yet neither is too much. Neither too much food nor not enough serves our health. As we study the extremes, we learn the power of the middle way. Between greed and scarcity is where abundance resides.

Between self-indulgence and severe asceticism is where Buddha found his middle way. We come to appreciate the creative possibility that lies in the realm between polar opposites. This appreciation is a step toward balance, freeing us from rigid thinking and attachment to extreme positions and allowing us to inhabit a center place of moderation and creativity. We move from a place of potential disequilibrium on either end of the teeter-totter to the center and equilibrium.

This is the place of balance, and balance is health. This is the place of accepting the whole, and wholeness is health. This is the terrain of the source of our healing power. This is deep medicine.

TOWARD A LIFE OF BALANCE AND WHOLENESS

We began our exploration of deep medicine with a description of the pursuit of health and healing as a lifelong quest for balance and wholeness requiring the capacity to change. The timeline of this quest is bounded by the bookends of birth and death. In between, the personal healing story of your life emerges in relationship to all that surrounds you. Your relationships connect you at all levels, from your atomic particles, cells, and organs to your family, loved ones, colleagues, and communities and ultimately to Mother Earth, the universe, and the unknowable. You are a separate entity and yet part of the whole, just as individual drops of water are part of the ocean's vastness, and each surface wave is inseparable from the deep, still waters beneath. The recognition and appreciation of the connection between the seen and unseen, the surface and the depths, the parts and the whole, the known and the unknowable reflect the connection between your outer and inner worlds. This defines the connection between the healing power that resides within you and those physical parts of your being with which and through which you uniquely present yourself to the outside world.

To your questions regarding health, illness, and well-being, there is no single answer. You have within you, as part of your human nature and your conditioning, a rich and varied potential for expression. No universal solution, recipe, protocol, or potion is available that, on its own, can take you to your desired destination. You exist within an extensive web of possibilities and can bring multiple points of view to bear when choosing among the endless options available to you. You must be willing to make your own way, set your own priorities, and accept the challenge of change. Your path will not be an unwavering straight line; it will involve stops and starts, backsliding, making unintended detours and even wrong turns, and, of course, it will involve life lessons and course corrections. You won't necessarily proceed through the stages of change in an orderly fashion or make use of all of the tools, pillars, and practices outlined in this book. You may spend a great deal of time on some and devote no time to others. You may explore other tools and practices or invent your own. Along the way, you will need both outside help and inner guidance. Much will depend on where you place your attention and the attitude and degree of vitality you bring to whatever you choose to do or not do.

From a scientific perspective, disease and illness are caused by biological and physical factors such as genetic makeup, environmental influences, and infectious agents. Healing practices, therefore, often use physical and technologic interventions. However, from a spiritual and mystical perspective, illness and suffering are universal aspects of life that require an awareness and form of understanding beyond the rational and scientific. Your inner healer deals with the forces of meaning, purpose, faith, belief, vulnerability, forgiveness, and love. You can make yourself sick, and you can create health. You can be creative and constructive, or you can be resistant and destructive. You have the capacity to be open and curious or to be judgmental and closed-minded. You can foster collaboration and practice compassion, and you can also be contrary, rigid, and arbitrary. You can bless and transgress. You are capable of laziness and procrastination. You can also create sacredness and beauty—and disorder. You can be filled with despair or hope. You can deny, be distracted, and get lost and broken, and in the very next moment you can choose to do something different.

Sometimes life will manifest in ways that are uplifting, generous, and kind. At other times you will be encased in grief, fatigue, or falsehood. You can find yourself in conflict and at war, or in peace, harmony, and contentment. You exist in a constantly changing reality that will require you to repeatedly make choices and changes to achieve, maintain, or regain your equilibrium. Much of your healing journey, and ultimately your health, will depend on your awareness, attention, attitude, and intentions. You must be willing to repeatedly assess your status and admit where you really are. Then you will need to act with authenticity, integrity, and honesty and take the next necessary step on your journey.

Your ability to identify, be in touch with, and act upon your states of being is deep medicine. This practice will reward you with a life of conscious awareness, clear thinking, compassionate feeling, and service-oriented action, all of which will be their own health-creating reward.

You have available, in what lies both within you and outside of you, exactly what you need to enhance your well-being. In everything you think, feel, say, and do, you have the capacity to be your own best medicine, anytime and everywhere.

FINDING BALANCE IN THE PRESENT MOMENT

A few years ago, I learned a valuable lesson in balance from a dear friend on a rocky beach surrounded by the natural beauty and grandeur of Flathead Lake in Montana. Sam had made his way to the shoreline early in the morning ahead of the rest of the group. There he had taken many river rocks the size of grapefruits and footballs and balanced them on top of each other.

How could those smooth-surfaced, rounded, heavy lumps be made to stand upright atop other, similar rocks? In most cases, only a small area of one rock was touching the one beneath, and their shapes were so irregular as to defy identifying them as geometric forms. Yet balance together at delicate points of contact they did.

Sam beckoned me as I watched his play, inviting me to try. As a child, I probably would have run, unbidden, to try it for myself. Yet as an adult I was hesitant. I was skeptical that it was possible to get those irregular lumps of stone aligned and upright—and concerned that I would fail. Cautiously, I eyed the balanced sculptures he was creating. Nervously, I lifted a rock and turned it over in my hands, looking for an appropriate facet on which to place it. The first one fell to the left. I repositioned it, seeking its preferred orientation. I set it again and again, gently adjusting and aligning it as it swayed and lurched in smaller arcs, my gestures ever smoother. Then, at one instant, it paused in perfect balance—unwavering and erect like a ballerina *en pointe*. I sighed, stepping back to admire my work.

Seconds later, a movement stimulated my peripheral vision and I looked up to see Risky Business, our host's exuberant Labrador retriever, bounding eagerly toward me and my precariously balanced sculpture. As his shiny, wet body knocked down my carefully constructed monument, I surprised myself by laughing. The shift created in my consciousness by having done something that seemed impossible was too big to be washed away by the transient nature of the accomplishment. I set off to find more rocks, discover their centers, and stand them up. With quiet, gentle attention, I found their subtle balance points—and mine.

Many times since, I have balanced rocks. The practice has been a quiet meditation, an inspiration, and a game. I have learned a great deal about balance—finding it, losing it, and finding it again. I have learned about impermanence and the transient nature of life, and about relationship—to myself, to the world around me, and to my work and companions.

In treating our illnesses and in creating our wellness, we are challenged to seek and maintain balance in our lives. As each of us struggles with our own unique path, we fashion our individual formulas and tools for well-being and healthy living. In so doing, we develop our special talents and then share them with those around us. As our individual gifts come together, we create healing for ourselves, our families, our communities, and, indeed, the entire planet.

TOWARD A NEW VISION OF HEALTH

Deep Medicine is a call to align your inner wisdom with what you are doing in the outside world in the pursuit of health and healing. As you develop your own practice of deep medicine, keep these important precepts in mind:

- All issues, in all domains of your life, are health issues.

- Everything you think, feel, say, and do is either health creating or health negating. Appreciating that everything impacts your health will allow you to build the connections between your well-being and your character, lifestyle choices, and relationships.

- To apply the principles of deep medicine, you must start by asking yourself the four questions of self-assessment in chapter 1: What am I thinking? What am I feeling? What am I doing? How is it working? Next, you must cultivate an internal, self-directed intention, willingness, and motivation to change. You must understand the stages and competencies for change, from chapter 2, and use the tools for change in chapter 3. You will have to commit to taking concrete action steps in all of the four pillars of self-care described in chapter 4; it isn't enough to think and talk about doing so. Most importantly, you must engage in the four practices described in chapter 4—slowing down, getting quiet, paying attention, and going inward—which will help you harness the source of your healing power. In particular, make use of the deep minute on a regular basis.

- You must see yourself, through your story, the stories of others, and the story of the planet, in the context of the bigger picture and greater good, not just in the context of your own self-interest. This connection from personal to planetary, my story to your story, and inner world to outer is about our belonging to all that is. Your external self, the player in the outside world, must partner with your inner power and healing wisdom for your health to truly flower and for complete healing to occur.

When you are able to slow down, get quiet, pay attention, and go inward, deep medicine will transform your life in ways that transcend simply healing your body. These skills will give you access to a rich health-creating resource, regardless of your circumstances and the issue at hand. And remember, the key is in what you do with the insights you gain. You can use the deep medicine ACTION plan below (Assess, Choose, Take steps, Integrate, Observe, and Negotiate) as a mnemonic to guide you in taking concrete steps on your personal healing path:

- **Assess:** Use the four questions of self-assessment to reflect on your life and how it is working for you.

- **Choose:** Decide whether a new course is warranted, and if so, choose to change.

- **Take steps:** Take the first bold step. Commit to health-creating behaviors, not merely thinking and talking about change.

- **Integrate:** Incorporate the new behaviors into your daily life through practice and repetition.

- **Observe:** Observe the results, make necessary course corrections, and then choose your next steps.

- **Negotiate:** Maintain ongoing negotiations with yourself and those closely involved with your health creation and healing, to ensure a healthful balance in your life.

It is possible to harness outer and inner sources of healing power and bring about a level of wellness that truly serves you, your loved ones, your community, and the planet. My hope is that Deep Medicine has given you renewable and sustainable tools to create your healing path, along with inspiring stories and motivation to be truly present and joyfully alive and well. My wish is that you develop your healing gifts and bring them to our evolving creation, contributing to your own well-being and the healing of the planet.

The winds of grace are always blowing,
but it is you that must raise your sail.

—Sri Ramakrishna

Resources

Following is an alphabetical listing of suggested readings. On my own path, I have drawn frequently from the works listed here. I am deeply grateful to the many teachers who have influenced my life. Look for audiotapes, CDs, and other works by the authors listed to further extend their teachings.

Achterberg, Jean. 1990. *Woman as Healer.* Boston: Shambhala.

Anderson, Robert A. 1987. *Wellness Medicine.* Lynnwood, WA: American Health Press.

Anderson, Robert A. 2001. *A Clinician's Guide to Holistic Medicine.* New York: Hazelden/McGraw-Hill.

Arrien, Angeles. 1992. *Signs of Life.* Sonoma, CA: Araus Publishing.

Arrien, Angeles. 1993. *The Four-Fold Way.* San Francisco: Harper.

Arrien, Angeles. 2000. *The Nine Muses: A Mythological Path to Creativity.* New York: Tarcher/Putnam.

Arrien, Angeles. 2005. *The Second Half of Life: Opening the Eight Gates of Wisdom.* Boulder, CO: Sounds True.

Artress, Lauren. 1995. *Walking a Sacred Path: Rediscovering the Labyrinth as a Spiritual Tool.* New York: Riverhead Books.

Baker, Dan, and Cameron Stauth. 2002. *What Happy People Know: How the New Science of Happiness Can Change Your Life for the Better*. Emmaus, PA: Rodale Books.

Balch, James, and Phyllis Balch. 1997. *Prescription for Nutritional Healing*. Garden City Park, NY: Avery Publishing Group.

Basu, Soumitra. 2000. *Integral Health: A Consciousness Approach to Health and Healing*. Pondicherry, India: Sri Aurobindo Ashram Press.

Bland, Jeffrey S., and Sara H. Benum. 1999. *Genetic Nutritioneering: How You Can Modify Inherited Traits and Live a Longer, Healthier Life*. Los Angeles: Keats Publishing.

Bolen, Jean Shinoda. 1996. *Close to the Bone*. New York: Scribner.

Boorstein, Sylvia. 2007. *Happiness Is an Inside Job*. New York: Ballantine Books.

Boorstein, Sylvia. 1996. *Don't Just Do Something, Sit There*. San Francisco: Harper.

Bridges, William. 1980. *Transitions*. New York: Addison-Wesley.

Cameron, Julia. 1992. *The Artist's Way: A Spiritual Path to Higher Creativity*. New York: Jeremy P. Tarcher/Putnam.

Cantwell, Michael. 2008. Map of the Spirit: Diagnosis and Treatment of Spiritual Disease. *Advances in Mind-Body Medicine* 23(2):6-17.

Capra, Fritjof. 1984. *The Tao of Physics*. New York: Bantam Books.

Chödrön, Pema. 1991. *The Wisdom of No Escape*. Boston: Shambhala.

Chödrön, Pema. 1994. *Start Where You Are*. Boston: Shambhala.

Chopra, Deepak. 1989. *Quantum Healing*. New York: Bantam Books.

Chopra, Deepak. 2000. *Perfect Health: The Complete Mind/Body Guide*. New York: Three Rivers Press.

Chopra, Deepak. 2004. *The Book of Secrets: Unlocking Hidden Dimensions of Your Life.* New York: Random House.

Coelho, Paulo. 1995. *The Pilgrimage.* San Francisco: Harper.

Coelho, Paulo. 1998. *The Alchemist.* New York: HarperCollins.

Cousins, Norman. 1979. *Anatomy of an Illness.* New York: W. W. Norton.

Dalai Lama and Howard C. Cutler. 1998. *The Art of Happiness.* New York: Riverhead Books.

Dass, Ram. 2000. *Still Here.* New York: Riverhead Books.

Dossey, Larry. 1999. *Reinventing Medicine.* San Francisco: Harper.

Douillard, John. 1994. *Body, Mind, and Spirit: The Mind-Body Guide to Lifelong Fitness and Your Personal Best.* New York: Crown.

Easwaran, Eknath. 2005. *Words to Live By: A Daily Guide to Leading an Exceptional Life.* Tomales, CA: Nilgiri Press.

Eisenberg, David M., Roger B. Davis, Susan L. Ettner, Scott Appel, Sonja Wilkey, Maria Van Rompay, and Ronald C. Kessler. 1998. Trends in Alternative Medicine Use in the United States, 1990-1997. *Journal of the American Medical Association* 280(18):1569-1575.

Fischer, Norman. 2008. *Sailing Home: Using the Wisdom of Homer's Odyssey to Navigate Life's Perils and Pitfalls.* New York: Free Press.

Fox, Matthew. 1991. *The Coming of the Cosmic Christ.* New York: Harper and Row.

Gardner, John W. 1995. *Self-Renewal: The Individual and the Innovative Society.* New York: W. W. Norton.

Gibran, Kahlil. 1989. *The Prophet.* New York: Alfred A. Knopf.

Goff, David. 1998. The Social Koan: Through Diversity to Interdependence. In A. Arrien (ed.), *Working Together: Producing*

Synergy by Honoring Diversity. Pleasanton, CA: New Leaders Press.

Golan, Ralph. 1995. *Optimal Wellness.* New York: Ballantine Books.

Gordon, James. 1996. *Manifesto for a New Medicine.* Reading, MA: Addison-Wesley.

Hanh, Thich Nhat. 1987. *The Miracle of Mindfulness.* Boston: Beacon Press.

Hobson, Charles. 1999. *Human Touch: Images for a Garden.* San Francisco: Pacific Editions.

Hora, Reenita Malhotra. 2004. *Inner Beauty.* San Francisco: Chronicle Books.

Irving, John. 1978. *The World According to Garp.* New York: E. P. Dutton.

Iyengar, B. K. S. 2001. *Yoga: The Path to Holistic Health.* London: Dorling Kindersley.

Iyengar, B. K. S. 2005. *Light on Life: The Yoga Journey to Wholeness, Inner Peace, and Ultimate Freedom.* Emmaus, PA: Rodale Books.

Kabat-Zinn, Jon. 1990. *Full Catastrophe Living.* New York: Dell Publishing.

Kabat-Zinn, Jon. 1994. *Wherever You Go, There You Are.* New York: Hyperion.

Kenny, Dennis K. 2002. *Promise of the Soul.* New York: John Wiley and Sons.

Kesten, Deborah. 2001. *The Healing Secrets of Food.* Novato, CA: New World Library.

Keyes, Ken, Jr. 1985. *The Hundredth Monkey.* Coos Bay, OR: Vision Books.

Kornfield, Jack. 1993. *A Path with Heart.* New York: Bantam Books.

Kornfield, Jack, and Christina Feldman. 1996. *Soul Food.* San Francisco: Harper.

Kula, Irwin. 2006. *Yearnings: Embracing the Sacred Messiness of Life.* New York: Hyperion.

Kushner, Lawrence. 1990. *The River of Light.* Woodstock, NY: Jewish Lights Publishing.

Lao Tzu. 1992. *Tao Te Ching.* Translated by Stephen Mitchell. New York: Harper Perennial/HarperCollins.

Lasater, Judith. 2000. *Living Your Yoga: Finding the Spiritual in Everyday Life.* Berkeley, CA: Rodmell Press.

Lele, Avinash, David Frawley, and Subhash Ranade. 2003. *Ayurveda and Marma Therapy: Energy Points in Yogic Healing.* Twin Lakes, WI: Lotus Press.

Levine, Stephen, and Ondrea Levine. 1982. *Who Dies?* New York: Anchor Books/Doubleday.

Liponis, Mark. 2007. *Ultra-Longevity: The Seven-Step Program for a Younger, Healthier You.* New York: Little Brown.

Loehe, Jim, and Tony Schwartz. 2003. *The Power of Full Engagement: Managing Energy, Not Time, Is the Key to High Performance and Personal Renewal.* New York: Free Press.

Longaker, Christine. 1997. *Facing Death and Finding Hope.* New York: Doubleday.

Lovelock, James. 1988. *The Ages of Gaia.* New York: Norton.

May, Rollo. 1975. *The Courage to Create.* New York: W. W. Norton.

Meade, Michael. 2005. *Fate and Destiny: The Eye of the Pupil, the Heart of the Disciple.* Audio CD. Seattle: Mosaic Voices.

Meade, Michael. 2005. *Fate and Destiny: The Two Agreements.* Audio CD. Seattle: Mosaic Voices.

Meyers, Norman (ed.). 1984. *Gaia: An Atlas of Planet Management.* New York: Anchor Books.

Muller, Wayne. 1996. *How Then Shall We Live? Four Simple Questions That Reveal the Beauty and Meaning of Our Lives.* New York: Bantam Books.

Muller, Wayne. 1999. *Sabbath: Restoring the Sacred Rhythm of Rest.* New York: Bantam Books.

Murray, Michael, and Joseph Pizzorno. 1998. *Encyclopedia of Natural Medicine.* Rocklin, CA: Prima Publishing.

Northrup, Christiane. 1998. *Women's Bodies, Women's Wisdom.* New York: Bantam Books.

O'Donohue, John. 1998. *Anam Cara: Spiritual Wisdom from the Celtic World.* New York: Cliff Street Books.

O'Donohue, John. 1999. *Eternal Echoes: Exploring Our Yearning to Belong.* New York: HarperCollins.

O'Donohue, John. 2007. *Benedictus: A Book of Blessings.* London: Transworld Publishers/Bantam Books.

O'Neill, Patrick. 1999. *Extraordinary Conversations.* 3 CD set. Toronto, Canada: Extraordinary Conversations.

Oman, Maggie (ed.). 1997. *Prayers for Healing.* Berkeley, CA: Conari Press.

Ornish, Dean. 1993. *Eat More, Weigh Less.* New York: HarperCollins.

Ornish, Dean. 1998. *Love and Survival.* New York: HarperCollins.

Oz, Mehmet, and Michael Roizen. 2007. *You: Staying Young. The Owner's Manual for Extending Your Warranty.* New York: Free Press. (Other books in this series are also useful resources.)

Patterson, Kerry, Joseph Grenny, Ron McMillan, and Al Switzler. 2002. *Crucial Conversations: Tools for Talking When Stakes Are High.* New York: McGraw-Hill.

Pelletier, Kenneth. 2000. *The Best Alternative Medicine: What Works? What Does Not?* New York: Simon and Schuster.

Prochaska, J., J. Norcross, and C. DiClemente. 1994. *Changing for Good: A Revolutionary Six-Stage Program for Overcoming Bad Habits and Moving Your Life Positively Forward.* New York: Avon Books.

Remen, Rachel Naomi. 1996. *Kitchen Table Wisdom.* New York: Riverhead Books.

Remen, Rachel Naomi. 2000. *My Grandfather's Blessings.* New York: Riverhead Books.

Rosenberg, Marshall. 2005. *Nonviolent Communication: A Language of Life.* Encinitas, CA: PuddleDancer Press.

Roszak, Theodore. 1992. *The Voice of the Earth.* New York: Simon and Schuster.

Rumi. 1995. *The Essential Rumi.* Translated by Coleman Barks. San Francisco: Harper.

Saint-Exupéry, Antoine de. 1971. *The Little Prince.* San Diego: Harcourt Brace.

Sapolsky, Robert M. 2001. *Why Zebras Don't Get Ulcers: An Updated Guide to Stress, Stress-Related Diseases, and Coping.* New York: N. H. Freeman and Co.

Scherwitz, Larry W., Michael Cantwell, Pamela McHenry, Claudia Wood, and William B. Stewart. 2004. A Descriptive Analysis of an Integrative Medicine Clinic. *Journal of Alternative and Complementary Medicine* 10(4):651-659.

Schiller, David (ed.). 1994. *The Little Zen Companion.* New York: Workman Publishing.

Schlitz, Marilyn, Tina Amorok, and Marc Micozzi. 2005. *Consciousness and Healing: Integral Approaches to Mind-Body Medicine.* St. Louis: Churchill Livingstone.

Sears, Barry, and Bill Lawren. 1995. *The Zone.* New York: HarperCollins.

Siegel, Bernie. 1988. *Love, Miracles and Medicine.* New York: Harper and Row.

Simopoulos, Artemis P., and Jo Robinson. 1999. *The Omega Diet.* New York: Harper Perennial.

Sobel, David, and Robert Ornstein. 1997. *The Healthy Mind, Healthy Body Handbook.* New York: Time-Life Books.

Sogyal Rinpoche. 1992. *The Tibetan Book of Living and Dying.* San Francisco: HarperCollins.

Spiegel, David. 1993. *Living Beyond Limits.* New York: Times Books/ Random House.

Stewart, William B. 1991. Physician Heal Thy Planet. *Western Journal of Medicine* 155(5):538-539.

Stewart, William B. 1993. Way of the Healer: The Work of Healing and the Healing of Work. *Western Journal of Medicine* 158(6):629-630.

Stewart, William B. 1994. Health Care: Transformation of Systems and Soul? *Western Journal of Medicine* 160(3):273-274.

Stewart, William B. 2000. The Institute for Health and Healing: Contributing to the Evolution of Contemporary Medicine. *San Francisco Medicine* 73(6):18-20.

Stewart, William B. 2000. Surgery, Service and Soul. *Ophthalmic Plastic and Reconstructive Surgery* 16(6):401-406.

Stewart, William B. 2001. Hospital-Based Integrative Medicine: The Institute for Health and Healing. In N. Faass (ed.), *Integrating Complementary Medicine into Health Systems*, pp. 406-411. Gaithersburg, MD: Aspen Publishers.

Stewart, William B. 2002. The Labyrinth: A Metaphoric Path to Health and Healing. *San Francisco Medicine* 75(5):23-25.

Stone, Douglas, Bruce Patton, and Sheila Heen. 2000. *Difficult Conversations: How to Discuss What Matters Most.* New York: Penguin Books.

Sun Tzu. 1991. *The Art of War.* Translated by Thomas Cleary. Boston: Shambhala.

Swimme, Brian, and Thomas Berry. 1992. *The Universe Story.* San Francisco: Harper.

Thomas, Lewis. 1974. *Lives of a Cell.* New York: Viking Press.

Thurston, Mark. 1987. *Paradox of Power.* Virginia Beach, VA: A.R.E. Press.

Thurston, Mark. 1989. *Soul-Purpose: Discovering and Fulfilling Your Destiny.* New York: St. Martin's Press.

Thurston, Mark. 2001. *Twelve Positive Habits of Spiritually Centered People.* Virginia Beach, VA: A.R.E. Press.

Tolle, Eckhart. 1999. *The Power of Now: A Guide to Spiritual Enlightenment.* Novato, CA: New World Library.

Tolle, Eckhart. 2006. *A New Earth: Awakening to Your Life's Purpose.* New York: Plume.

Venkataswamy, Govindappa. 1994. *Illuminated Spirit.* New York: Paulist Press.

Venkataswamy, Govindappa. 2004. *Infinite Vision.* DVD. Directed by Pavithra Krishnan. Madurai, India: Aravind Eye Care System.

Watson, Lyall. 1980. *Lifetide.* New York: Simon and Schuster.

Watts, Alan. 1951. *The Wisdom of Insecurity.* New York: Vintage Books/Random House.

Webb, Wyatt, with Cindy Pearlman. 2002. *It's Not About the Horse— It's About Overcoming Fear and Self-Doubt.* Carlsbad, CA: Hay House.

Weil, Andrew. 1997. *Eight Weeks to Optimum Health.* New York: Alfred A. Knopf.

Weil, Andrew. 2000. *Eating Well for Optimum Health.* New York: Alfred A. Knopf.

Weil, Andrew. 2005. *Healthy Aging.* New York: Alfred A. Knopf.

White, Timothy. 1993. *The Wellness Guide to Lifelong Fitness.* New York: Rebus.

Wilber, Ken. 2000. *The Theory of Everything.* Boston: Shambhala.

Zukav, Gary. 1989. *The Dancing Wu Li Masters.* New York: Bantam Books.

References

Achterberg, J. 1990. *Woman as Healer*. Boston: Shambhala.

Annas, G. J. 1995. Reframing the debate on health care reform by replacing our metaphors. *New England Journal of Medicine* 332(11):745-748.

Arrien, A. 1993. *The Four-Fold Way*. San Francisco: Harper.

Arrien, A. 2005. *The Second Half of Life: Opening the Eight Gates of Wisdom*. Boulder, CO: Sounds True.

Artress, L. 1995. *Walking a Sacred Path: Rediscovering the Labyrinth as a Spiritual Tool*. New York: Riverhead Books.

Astin, J. 1998. Why patients use alternative medicine. *Journal of the American Medical Association* 279(19):1548-1553.

Baker, D., and C. Stauth. 2002. *What Happy People Know: How the New Science of Happiness Can Change Your Life for the Better*. Emmaus, PA: Rodale Books.

Bland, J. S., and S. H. Benum. 1999. *Genetic Nutritioneering: How You Can Modify Inherited Traits and Live a Longer, Healthier Life*. Los Angeles: Keats Publishing.

Boorstein, S. 2007. *Happiness Is an Inside Job*. New York: Ballantine Books.

Browner, W. S., A. J. Kahn, E. Ziv, A. P. Reiner, J. Oshima, R. M. Cawthon, W. C. Hsueh, and S. R. Cummings. 2004. The Genetics of Human Longevity. *American Journal of Medicine* 117(11):851-860.

Capra, F. 1984. *The Tao of Physics*. New York: Bantam Books.

Center for Ecoliteracy. 2008. Principles of Ecology. www.ecoliteracy. org/education/principles_of_ecology.html.

Chopra, D., D. Ornish, R. Roy, and A. Weil. 2009. "Alternative" medicine is mainstream. *Wall Street Journal* January 9, 2009.

Cohen, J. T., P. J. Neumann, and M. C. Weinstein. 2008. Does preventive care save money? Health economics and the presidential candidates. *New England Journal of Medicine* 358(7):661-663.

Cousineau, P. 1998. *The Art of Pilgrimage*. Berkeley, CA: Conari Press.

Cousins, N. 1979. *Anatomy of an Illness*. New York: W. W. Norton.

Dass, Ram. 1990. *Journey of Awakening: A Meditator's Guidebook*. New York: Bantam.

Easwaran, E. (trans.). 2000. *The Bhagavad Gita*. New York: Vintage Books.

Eyre, H., R. Kahn, R. M. Robertson, N. G. Clark, C. Doyle, Y. Hong, T. Gansler, T. Glynn, R. A. Smith, K. Taubert, and M. J. Thun. 2004. Preventing cancer, cardiovascular disease, and diabetes: A common agenda for the American Cancer Society, the American Diabetes Association, and the American Heart Association. *Circulation* 109(25):3244-3255.

Gallia, K. 2001. America's healthiest hospitals. *Natural Health*, December, 58.

Golden, H. 1958. *Only in America*. Cleveland, OH: World Publishing.

Kleinman, A. 1981. *Patients and Healers in the Context of Culture: An Exploration of the Borderland Between Anthropology, Medicine, and Psychiatry.* Berkeley: University of California Press.

Kleinman, A., L. Eisenberg, and B. Good. 1978. Culture, illness, and care: Clinical lessons from anthropologic and cross-cultural research. *Annals of Internal Medicine* 88(2)251-258.

Kornfield, J. 1993. *A Path with Heart.* New York: Bantam Books.

Liester, M. B. 1996. Inner voices: Distinguishing transcendent and pathological characteristics. *Journal of Transpersonal Psychology* 28(1):14.

Luther, M., H. E. Jacobs, and A. Spaeth. 1930. *Works of Martin Luther: With Introductions and Notes,* vol. 3. Philadelphia: A. J. Holman and the Castle Press.

Malik, S., N. D. Wong, S. S. Franklin, T. V. Kamath, G. J. L'Italien, J. R. Pio, and G. R. Williams. 2004. Impact of the metabolic syndrome on mortality from coronary heart disease, cardiovascular disease, and all causes in United States adults. *Circulation* 110(10):1245-1250.

Marshall, P. H. 1996. *Nature's Web: Rethinking Our Place on Earth.* Armonk, NY: M. E. Sharpe.

Maslow, A. 1999. *Toward a Psychology of Being.* New York: John Wiley and Sons.

Miller, W. R., and J. C'deBaca. 1994. Quantum change: Toward a psychology of transformation. In T. Heatheron and J. Weinberger (eds.), *Can Personality Change?* pp. 253-280. Washington, DC: American Psychological Association.

Miller, W. R., and S. Rollnick. 2002. *Motivational Interviewing: Preparing People for Change.* New York: Guilford Press.

Mills, B., with N. Sparks. 1999. *Wokini: A Lakota Journey to Happiness and Self-Understanding.* Carlsbad, CA: Hays House.

Myss, C. 1997. *Why People Don't Heal and How They Can.* New York: Harmony Books.

O'Donohue, J. 1998. *Anam Cara: Spiritual Wisdom from the Celtic World.* New York: Cliff Street Books.

O'Neil, G., and G. O'Neil. 1990. *The Human Life.* Spring Valley, NY: Mercury Press.

Ornish, D., J. Lin, J. Daubenmier, G. Weidner, E. Epel, C. Kemp, M. J. M. Magbaunua, R. Marlin, L. Yglecias, P. R. Carroll, and E. H. Blackburn. 2008. Increased telomerase activity and comprehensive lifestyle changes: A pilot study. *Lancet Oncology* 9(11):1048-1057.

Prochaska, James, John Norcross, and Carlo DiClemente. 1994. *Changing for Good: A Revolutionary Six-Stage Program for Overcoming Bad Habits and Moving Your Life Positively Forward.* New York: Avon Books.

Robinson, B. H. 2007. *Biomedicine: A Textbook for Practitioners of Acupuncture and Oriental Medicine.* Boulder, CO: Blue Poppy Press.

Sogyal Rinpoche. 1992. *The Tibetan Book of Living and Dying.* San Francisco: HarperCollins.

Sun Tzu. 1991. *The Art of War.* Translated by Thomas Cleary. Boston: Shambhala.

Swimme, B., and T. Berry. 1992. *The Universe Story.* San Francisco: Harper.

Venkataswamy, G. 2004. *Infinite Vision.* DVD. Directed by Pavithra Krishnan. Madurai, India: Aravind Eye Care System.

Webb, W., with C. Pearlman. 2002. *It's Not About the Horse—It's About Overcoming Fear and Self-Doubt.* Carlsbad, CA: Hay House.

Zukav, G. 1989. *The Dancing Wu Li Masters.* New York: Bantam Books.

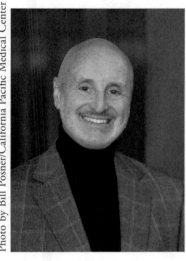

William B. Stewart, MD, is cofounder and medical director of the Institute for Health and Healing at the California Pacific Medical Center in San Francisco. He has been voted by his peers as one of the best doctors in America for many years through the Best Doctors, Inc., organization. Dr. Stewart's work has been informed by medical volunteer work in India and more than thirty years of surgical practice. His personal experiences have contributed to a profound perspective on the cycles of life and the principles and practices of mindful living. For more information about *Deep Medicine*, Dr. Stewart, or the Institute for Health and Healing, visit www.myhealthandhealing.org.

Foreword writer **Angeles Arrien, Ph.D.,** is a cultural anthropologist, educator, and consultant to many organizations and businesses. She lectures and conducts workshops worldwide on cultural anthropology, psychology, and comparative religion. Arrien is president of the Foundation for Cross-Cultural Education and Research. Her books have been translated into nine languages, and she has received three honorary doctorate degrees in recognition of her work. Angeles Arrien lives in the San Francisco Bay area.

About the Institute of Noetic Sciences (IONS)

Noetic Books is an imprint of the Institute of Noetic Sciences, which was founded in 1973 by Apollo 14 astronaut Edgar Mitchell. IONS is a 501(c)(3) nonprofit research, education, and membership organization whose mission is advancing the science of consciousness and human experience to serve individual and collective transformation. "Noetic" comes from the Greek word *nous*, which means "intuitive mind" or "inner knowing." The Institute's primary program areas include consciousness and healing, extended human capacities, and emerging worldviews. The specific work of the institute includes the following:

- Sponsorship of and participation in original research

- Publication of the quarterly magazine *Shift: At the Frontiers of Consciousness*

- The monthly membership program, Shift in Action, and its associated website, www.shiftinaction.com

- Presentation and cosponsorship of regional and international workshops and conferences

- The hosting of residential seminars and workshops at its on-campus retreat facility, located on 200 acres thirty minutes north of San Francisco

- The support of a global volunteer network of community groups

IONS also publishes *The Shift Report*, a now bi-annual publication that charts shifts in worldview across a wide range of disciplines and areas of human activity. Information on these reports can be found at *www.shiftreport.org*. More information about Noetic Books is available at *www.noeticbooks.org*.

To learn more about the Institute and its activities and programs, please contact

Institute of Noetic Sciences
101 San Antonio Road
Petaluma, CA 94952-9524
707-775-3500 / fax: 707-781-7420
www.noetic.org

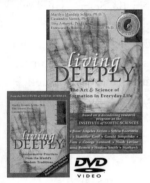
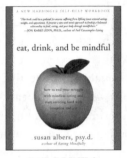
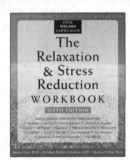
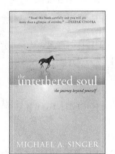
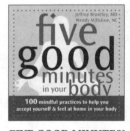
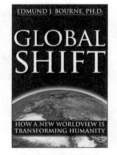